Chronic Pain

About the Authors

Beverly J. Field, PhD, is Assistant Professor in the Departments of Anesthesiology and Psychiatry, Washington University School of Medicine, St. Louis, Missouri. She is cofounder and director of the STEPP program, a cognitive-behavioral program for patients with chronic pain. In addition to her clinical and teaching responsibilities, she lectures regularly on psychological therapies in multidisciplinary pain management.

Robert A. Swarm, MD, is Associate Professor and Chief, Division of Pain Management in the Department of Anesthesiology, Washington University School of Medicine, St. Louis, Missouri. He is also the Director of the Pain Management Fellowship Training Program at Washington University, and Director of the Barnes-Jewish Hospital, Washington University Pain Management Center. His clinical work is exclusively focused on the multidisciplinary management of acute, chronic, and cancer pain.

Dr. Field and Dr. Swarm have been colleagues at the Barnes-Jewish Hospital, Washington University Pain Management Center since 1994.

Advances in Psychotherapy – Evidence-Based Practice

Danny Wedding; PhD, MPH, Prof., St. Louis, MO
(Series Editor)
Larry Beutler; PhD, Prof., Palo Alto, CA
Kenneth E. Freedland; PhD, Prof., St. Louis, MO
Linda C. Sobell; PhD, ABPP, Prof., Ft. Lauderdale, FL
David A. Wolfe; PhD, Prof., Toronto
(Associate Editors)

The basic objective of this series is to provide therapists with practical, evidence-based treatment guidance for the most common disorders seen in clinical practice – and to do so in a "reader-friendly" manner. Each book in the series is both a compact "how-to-do" reference on a particular disorder for use by professional clinicians in their daily work, as well as an ideal educational resource for students and for practice-oriented continuing education.

The most important feature of the books is that they are practical and "reader-friendly:" All are structured similarly and all provide a compact and easy-to-follow guide to all aspects that are relevant in real-life practice. Tables, boxed clinical "pearls", marginal notes, and summary boxes assist orientation, while checklists provide tools for use in daily practice.

Chronic Pain

Beverly J. Field
Washington University School of Medicine, St. Louis, MO

Robert A. Swarm
Washington University School of Medicine, St. Louis, MO

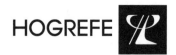

Library of Congress Cataloging in Publication

is available via the Library of Congress Marc Database under the
LC Control Number 2007938384

Library and Archives Canada Cataloguing in Publication

Field, Beverly J
    Chronic pain / Beverly J. Field, Robert A. Swarm.   .

(Advances in psychotherapy–evidence-based practice)
Includes bibliographical references.
ISBN 978-0-88937-320-4

    1. Chronic pain–Psychological aspects. 2. Chronic pain–Treatment.
I. Swarm, Robert A. II. Title. III. Series.

RB127.F44 2008   616'.0472019   C2007-906047-1

PUBLISHING OFFICES
USA: Hogrefe & Huber Publishers, 875 Massachusetts Avenue, 7th Floor,
                 Cambridge, MA 02139
                 Phone (866) 823-4726, Fax (617) 354-6875; E-mail info@hhpub.com
EUROPE: Hogrefe & Huber Publishers, Rohnsweg 25, 37085 Göttingen, Germany
                 Phone +49 551 49609-0, Fax +49 551 49609-88, E-mail hh@hhpub.com

SALES & DISTRIBUTION
USA: Hogrefe & Huber Publishers, Customer Services Department,
                 30 Amberwood Parkway, Ashland, OH 44805
                 Phone (800) 228-3749, Fax (419) 281-6883, E-mail custserv@hhpub.com
EUROPE: Hogrefe & Huber Publishers, Rohnsweg 25, 37085 Göttingen, Germany
                 Phone +49 551 49609-0, Fax +49 551 49609-88, E-mail hh@hhpub.com

OTHER OFFICES
CANADA: Hogrefe & Huber Publishers, 1543 Bayview Avenue, Toronto, Ontario M4G 3B5
SWITZERLAND: Hogrefe & Huber Publishers, Länggass-Strasse 76, CH-3000 Bern 9

Hogrefe & Huber Publishers
Incorporated and registered in the State of Washington, USA, and in Göttingen, Lower Saxony,
Germany

Printed and bound in the USA
ISBN 978-0-88937-320-4

Foreword

Chronic pain is highly prevalent with one third of Americans experiencing frequent or persistent pain. Of those who have pain, function or quality of life is significantly impacted. Chronic pain is also extraordinarily complex, at times associated with progressive damage to virtually any tissue, or occurring in the absence of an explanatory lesion. Some patients are highly disabled by their pain, whereas others function well despite similar pathology.

From a clinical perspective, it is useful to classify pain as nociceptive or neuropathic pain, acute or chronic, cancer or noncancer, in the back or in the abdomen. Classification leads to treatment guidelines and best practices yet these distinctions are an extreme simplification. Chronic pain is better understood as the integration of related processes – biomedical and psychological – that may sustain pain and predispose individuals. Chronic pain is, in fact, many diseases only now being defined, classified, and analyzed. For many patients chronic pain becomes the disease itself with the sensory experience of pain and the adverse effects on mood and function. This understanding of pain as illness is one of the foundations of the modern approach to pain management.

There is substantial documentation that many, if not the majority of patients suffering pain remain vastly underdiagnosed and undertreated. Even with evidence-based consensus, best-practice approaches are not being followed for most patients, and access to specialists is very limited. Chronic pain has become a major public health problem with annual costs in the United States estimated at $100 billion.

Chronic Pain presents up-to-date information to the provider who has been overlooked in the treatment of pain. In the attempt to look for pathology and treat symptoms, the role of psychology has been underestimated. Any chronic illness is best treated with a patient-focused, integrated approach relying heavily on patient self-care. Patients need to learn management skills, controlling symptoms while maintaining meaningful and active lifestyles. Psychology is uniquely positioned to help in this treatment. This volume joins an ever-growing number of books, journals, and other sources of information that document these advances and educate the health care giver about pain and its management.

Progress comes slowly and treatment can be controversial. The debate often reaches into the area of public policy with mandated pain education and prosecution of providers for over- and underprescribing of opioids. Nonetheless, the advances in research and the increasing number of consensus views within the professional community provide the means to help many patients. Pain is complex and ever-changing. Treating patients requires time and patience. Perhaps it will someday be possible that every patient will have access to competent care for the potentially devastating illness of chronic pain.

Bill H. McCarberg, MD
Chronic Pain Management Program, Kaiser Permanente, San Diego
School of Medicine, University of California, San Diego

Table of Contents

1

Description of the Disorder

1.1   Definitions

Pain is a basic biological warning mechanism signaling tissue damage and physiological harm. It was described by Albert Schweitzer (1931, p. 62) as "…a more terrible Lord of mankind than even death itself." In *Paradise Lost*, Milton (1910, p. 47) wrote that, "Pain is perfect misery, the worst of evils, and excessive, overturns all patience." Webster's dictionary (1983) defines pain as: (1) The sensations one feels when hurt mentally or physically, especially distress, suffering, great anxiety, anguish, grief, etc.: opposed to pleasure. (2) A sensation of hurting or strong discomfort in some part of the body. These descriptions and definitions speak to both the sensation of pain and to the suffering that accompanies it.

Pain is a complex, subjective experience with no objective tests or physiological markers

The International Association for the Study of Pain Subcommittee on Taxonomy (Mersky, 1979) defined pain as:

> An unpleasant sensory and emotional experience associated with actual or potential tissue damage, or described in terms of such damage.

This definition recognizes the complexity of pain, its sensory and emotional aspects, and its subjective nature. There are no reliable tests or consistent physiological markers of pain, and it is not always referable to any objective findings. To understand another person's pain, it is necessary to rely on the subjective narration of his or her personal experience. The subjectivity of pain is acknowledged in the International Association for the Study of Pain (IASP) definition, as is the recognition of pain in the absence of tissue damage, which discounts previously held distinctions between somatogenic (or "real") pain and psychogenic (or "imaginary") pain.

1.2   Terminology

It will be helpful to have a working knowledge of pain-related terminology and classifications. Some of the more common terms are listed below. A more comprehensive list of terms may be found in Mersky and Bogduk's *Classification of Chronic Pain* (1994).

Table 1
Terminology and Definitions

Term	Definition
Allodynia	Pain resulting from a stimulus that would normally not produce pain, such as a light touch or a breeze.
Analgesia	Absence of pain in response to stimulation that would normally be painful.
Central pain	Pain initiated or caused by a lesion or dysfunction in the spinal cord or brain.
Hyperalgesia	Increased sensitivity to a stimulus that is normally painful.
Hypoalgesia	Diminished sensitivity to a stimulus that is normally painful.
Neuralgia	Pain in the distribution of a nerve.
Neuropathy	A disturbance of function or pathological change in one or more nerves.
Nociceptor	A receptor preferentially receptive to a noxious stimulus.
Noxious stimulus	A stimulus that is damaging to normal tissue.
Pain threshold	The lowest stimulus intensity at which a person can recognize pain.
Pain tolerance	The greatest stimulus intensity causing pain that a person is prepared to tolerate.

1.2.1   Classification of Pain

Pain may be classified along various dimensions, the most common of which are:

- Temporal (acute, chronic, and episodic)
- Mechanism of transmission (nociceptive, neuropathic, central)
- Disease state causing the pain (arthritis, diabetic neuropathy)
- Anatomical site (low back pain, neck or knee pain)

Temporal

Acute pain is one of the most frequent reasons for seeking medical care

Acute pain is of brief duration, generally less than six months, and is usually associated with tissue damage. In the case of injury, acute pain is an adaptive and necessary biological signal of tissue damage and physiological harm. It serves to increase awareness and calls for an action or response such as withdrawing a limb from danger. In most cases of acute pain, the cause is known and adequate treatment is available. When healing is complete, the pain resolves. The initial emotional responses to acute pain, such as fear and anxiety, can serve to motivate care seeking and limitation of movement. Examples of acute pain include bony fractures, sprains, puncture wounds, childbirth, various acute disease states, and postsurgical pain.

Chronic pain persists for an extended period of time. It is usually defined as pain lasting longer than six months or pain that persists beyond the expected time for healing. Unlike acute pain, the signal of chronic pain does not serve as a warning of further tissue damage and generally serves no adaptive purpose.

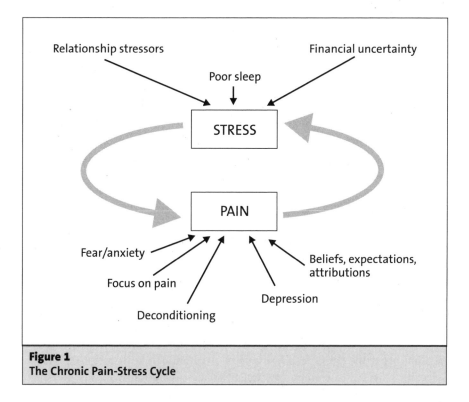

Figure 1
The Chronic Pain-Stress Cycle

The cause or causes of chronic pain may or may not be known in any given case. If the cause is known, it may or may not be amenable to a cure. Chronic pain interferes with normal functioning and daily living, and can be detrimental to overall health. It is often associated with loss of employment, inability to participate in recreational activities, financial distress, and changes in relationships, personal identity, and feelings of self-worth. Chronic pain is often referred to as chronic noncancer pain, in distinction from cancer pain, which may be caused by tumor invasion into tissue, obstruction of organs, compression or infiltration of nerves, painful procedures, or antitumor therapies such as radiation or chemotherapy.

   In the transition from acute to chronic pain, psychological factors play a changing and increasingly important role in pain perception and coping. Chronic pain is complex, and is associated with changes in physiological responses, dysphoric mood states such as depression, helplessness, guilt, and apathy, increased preoccupation with pain, and a general eroding of internal resources. In addition, chronic pain is accompanied by a multitude of behavioral responses including severely restricted activity, sleep deprivation, and social withdrawal. Examples of chronic noncancer pain include chronic low back pain, postherpetic neuralgia after shingles, osteoarthritis, and fibromyalgia.

   Recurrent, intermittent, or episodic pain is acute, in that each episode is of limited duration, but also chronic in that the episodes occur over a period of time lasting longer than six months. Although persons with episodic pain do not suffer from pain continuously, repeated episodes of pain may disrupt normal functioning at school, work and/or in personal relationships. Examples of episodic pain include migraine headache and sickle cell crises.

Chronic pain is now recognized as an independent disease state

Throughout this manual, references to pain will mean chronic noncancer pain unless otherwise noted. Although acute, cancer, and episodic pain present their own unique challenges, it is the extended time frame of chronic pain that brings about the life changes and emotional responses that result in its complexity and resistance to management.

Neurophysiology of Pain Signal Transmission

Nociception is the process of detection and transmission of pain signals from the site of injury to the central nervous system (CNS). The details of how nerve signals are transmitted, and ultimately perceived as pain, are not fully understood, although several processes are known to underlie nociception. In the process of transduction, energy from a noxious stimulus (thermal, mechanical, or chemical) is converted into nerve impulses by receptors called nociceptors. These nerve impulses, or pain signals, are then transmitted from the site of injury to the spinal cord and brain. The signals or nerve impulses are perceived as pain after reaching the brain. Pain signal transmission is continuously modulated by factors that either facilitate or inhibit transmission throughout the nervous system.

> **Signal transmission from injury does not result in pain until the information reaches the brain**

Nociceptive pain results from tissue damage, the source of which may be mechanical, thermal, or chemical. Nociceptive pain occurs when pain-specific neurons are activated in response to noxious stimulation. Nociceptors are specifically sensitive to pain-enhancing substances associated with inflammation. Depending on its etiology, nociceptive pain may be described as dull and aching, sharp and burning, or cramping and pulling. Examples of nociceptive pain include: burns, cuts, and bruises, bony fractures, appendicitis, and pancreatitis.

The processes of pain signal transduction, transmission, and perception are dynamic and may vary greatly within an individual over time, as well as between individuals. Factors that may facilitate pain signal transduction and transmission include nociceptor activity itself (due to positive feedback mechanisms), tissue injury and inflammation, damage to nerves as in neuropathic pain (see below), and chronic opioid use (opioid tolerance hyperalgesia). Inflammation, which induces the swelling and erythema that are often associated with tissue injury, is an integral component of the normal tissue response to injury that leads to healing. Inflammation also markedly affects the function of nociceptors to facilitate the transduction and transmission of pain signals. Inflammation-induced facilitation of nociceptor function is one of the principal causes for the extreme severity of pain associated with tissue injury (e.g., surgery), infection (e.g., boils), and inflammatory disease (rheumatoid arthritis).

> **Factors that facilitate/inhibit pain transmission can influence sensation and/or unpleasantness**

Hyperalgesia, an increased response to normally noxious (painful) stimuli, and allodynia, the perception as painful of normally nonnoxious stimuli, are common clinical findings that suggest the activation of mechanisms of pain signal facilitation. In many cases in which a person seems to be experiencing pain "out of proportion to that expected," the explanation lies not in undiagnosed psychopathology but in mechanisms of neural facilitation of pain signal transduction/transmission.

Neuropathic pain results from damage to a peripheral nerve or to dysfunction in the central nervous system, and it often occurs in the absence of ongoing tissue damage. A remarkable example is phantom limb pain, in which pain continues despite the absence of the physical structure, e.g., phantom pain in

Table 2
Disorders and Treatments Associated with Neuropathic Pain

Diabetes

Herpes zoster (shingles)

Spinal cord injury

Cancer
    Chemo- or radiation therapy
    Tumor compression or infiltration of nerves

Complex Regional Pain Syndrome
    Type I (reflex sympathetic dystrophy)
    Type II (causalgia)

Limb amputation

Multiple sclerosis

Stroke, especially those involving the thalamus

Trigeminal neuralgia

HIV infection

Sciatica

Trauma with injury to peripheral nerves

the "hand" of an amputated arm. In phantom limb pain, the nervous system continues to generate pain signals perceived as pain in the missing limb. Neuropathic pain can result from direct damage to nerves such as from cutting, stretching, or crushing injuries, inflammation, pressure (such as may result from tumor infiltration), or compression or entrapment by damaged spinal disks, joints, or scar tissue.

Neuropathic pain is usually described as sharp, shooting, burning, or lancinating (stabbing) and is often associated with abnormal sensations such as "electrical shocks" or "pins and needles." The presence of chronic hyperalgesia, and/or allodynia, in the absence of tissue injury or inflammation, should raise the suspicion that nerve injury or disease (i.e., neuropathy) is the cause of the pain.

Common Disease States Associated with Chronic Pain

Arthritis. The term arthritis refers to over one hundred conditions, the best known being osteo- and rheumatoid arthritis. Arthritis is not curable, but is often manageable with patient education, medical management, and nonpharmacologic treatment.

Osteoathritis, also called degenerative joint disease, most commonly affects older adults although it can develop in younger individuals following injury or with repetitive stress. In osteoarthritis, the cartilage, which protects bone and allows joints to move easily, becomes damaged through persistent low-grade inflammation and degeneration. The cartilage damage results in bones rubbing against one another, causing pain and swelling. Osteoarthritis most frequently affects weight-bearing joints and can result from excessive

Obesity is associated with knee pain and hip osteoarthritis

loading-bearing activities, obesity, or aging. Osteoarthritis commonly affects the feet, ankles, knees, hips, low back, neck, and fingers. It is experienced as stiffness, particularly in the morning, which usually improves with movement. Pain can increase over the course of the day with weight bearing and activity. Treatment for osteoarthritis includes: patient education; cognitive behavioral approaches; low-impact physical therapy aimed at improving flexibility, range of motion, muscle conditioning, and aerobic fitness; weight loss (in obese patients); medications (acetaminophen and nonsteroidal anti-inflammatory drugs [NSAIDs]); cortisone injections; use of assistive devices (canes, crutches, walkers); pain medication; topical treatments (heat, ice, menthol and capsaicin ointments), and surgery.

Rheumatoid arthritis is a systemic inflammatory disease. It is a chronic autoimmune disorder that begins with inflammation in the lining of the joint. The inflamed joint fluid produces a chemical response, which results in destruction of bone and cartilage. Manifestations of rheumatoid arthritis include pain, swelling, warmth, and tenderness in affected joints. The joint damage often leads to loss of function and disability.

Rheumatoid arthritis affects more women than men, in a ratio of 5:1 (Simon et al., 2002). Although the onset of rheumatoid arthritis generally occurs between the ages of 30 and 50, children can be affected by juvenile rheumatoid arthritis. Rheumatoid arthritis should be treated early and aggressively in an effort to limit permanent joint damage. Treatment for rheumatoid arthritis includes: medications (disease-modifying antirheumatic drugs [DMARDs], acetaminophen, and NSAIDs); patient education; cognitive behavioral approaches; low-impact physical therapy to improve flexibility and range of motion, muscle strength, and aerobic conditioning; weight loss (in obese patients); cortisone injections; use of assistive devices (canes, crutches, walkers); pain medications; topical treatments (heat, ice, menthol and capsaicin ointments), and surgery.

Fibromyalgia is a chronic pain syndrome accompanied by widespread tenderness, poor sleep, fatigue, cognitive dysfunction, and emotional distress. The criteria specified by the American College of Rheumatology for a diagnosis of fibromyalgia include: (a) a history of widespread pain and (b) excessive tenderness in at least 11 of 18 muscle-tendon sites (Burckhardt et al., 2005). Fibromyaglia is a syndrome, not a disease, and the cause is not known. It is associated with other features such as headache, disrupted and/or nonrestorative sleep, chronic fatigue, and irritable bowel syndrome. Current research suggests that fibromyalgia may be a pain syndrome of the central nervous system that includes aberrant pain signal transmission and pain processing. It is more prevalent in women than in men. Treatment includes education, medications, sleep hygiene, slowly progressive low-impact exercises, stress reduction, trigger point injections, and coping skills training.

Anatomical Sites

Low back pain is common in industrialized countries. It is one of the most frequent presenting complaints among people seeking primary medical care, second only to symptoms of the common cold. In the United States, back disorders are the leading cause of worker disability. These disorders are associated with high direct costs such as medical care and disability payments, and indirect costs such as lost wages and diminished productivity. Approximately

The Arthritis Foundation can be an excellent patient resource

Excellent sources of information are the Clinical Practice Guidelines published by the APS

Low back pain is one of the primary causes of absence from work

70–85% of adults will experience at least one episode of low back pain during their lifetime. Most will recover within one month with 80–90% showing recovery without functional loss within 12 weeks. However, of patients disabled from back pain longer than 6 months, fewer than half return to work and, after 2 years of absence from work due to low back pain, the return to work rate approaches zero (Andersson, 1999). In 85% of these cases, the cause of the back pain is unknown (Deyo & Weinstein, 2001). Low back pain can arise from numerous sources including:

- Muscle tightness (spasm)
- Muscle or ligament strain or tear
- Degeneration, herniation, or rupture of the intervertebral disks
- Narrowing of the spinal canal (spinal stenosis)
- Fractures of the spine due to osteoporosis
- Abnormal curvature of the spine (scoliosis or kyphosis)
- Infection
- Trauma

1.3   Epidemiology

1.3.1   Prevalence of Chronic Pain

It is difficult to obtain accurate epidemiological data on the prevalence, severity, and impact of chronic pain. Because there are no objective tests for pain, and because self-reported pain is subjective, it is often difficult to obtain consensus about whether or not a specific condition is present. Classification of low back pain could be based on objective findings, such as disk herniation on MRI, or on functional status and disability. The use of one or the other, or both classifications, would influence prevalence rates. Of cases of low back pain in the general population, it has been reported that as many as 85% have no objective findings. On the other hand, many individuals with abnormal findings on spinal imaging deny having any back pain. The multiple dimensions of chronic pain conditions lead to highly diverse presentations of its biological, psychological, and social components. In addition, multiple disease states and syndromes often contribute to the larger picture of chronic pain.

The prevalence of chronic pain is the proportion of individuals with chronic pain at a specified period of time

In spite of these limitations, epidemiologic surveys undertaken over the past 30 years have identified the prevalence, risk factors, and management of chronic pain. In Western countries, prevalence estimates of chronic pain in the general population range from 10% to 55%, with slightly higher rates among females (Harstall & Ospina, 2003). Approximately 70 million Americans report chronic pain, with 10% having pain for more than 100 days per year (Von Korff & LeResche, 2005).

Second only to colds and flu, pain is the foremost reason for visits to physicians

1.3.2   Economic Impact of Pain

Chronic pain exacts tremendous costs from patients, employers, and the health care system. A study by Stewart, Ricci, Chee, Morganstein, and Lipton (2003)

Table 3
Period Prevalence Rates (One Year or Less) of Common Chronic Pain Conditions in Adults.

Pain Condition	Median Prevalence Estimate (%)	Range of Prevalence Estimates (No. Studies)	Sex Differences in Prevalence Rates
Headache	69% in females 46% in males	3–99% (F) 3–93% (M) (33 studies)	More common in women
Low back pain	37%	10–63% (11 studies)	No differences by sex in most studies
Knee pain	18%	10–29% (11 studies)	More common among women but sex differences reduced at older ages
Neck pain	16% in females 12% in males	10–40% (F) 3–29% (M) (4 studies)	More common in women
Migraine	15% in females 6% in males	10–40% (F) 0–46% (M) (32 studies)	More common among women
Chronic wide-spread pain	8%	0.66–10.7% (8 studies)	More common in women
Temporo-mandibular pain	9% in females 5% in males	5–14% (F) 3–10% (M) (10 studies)	More common in women
Shoulder pain	7%	2–61% (5 studies)	Sex difference are inconsistent

From Von Korff, M., & LeResche, L. Epidemiology of Pain. In: Merskey H., Loeser, J. D., & Dubner, R. (2005) (Eds.). The Paths of Pain 1975-2005. IASP Press: Seattle. Page 341, used with permission.

Chronic pain is not itself curable

used data from the American Productivity Audit, from August 2001 to July 2002, to estimate productivity losses to employers over a two-week period. They estimated that 13% of the work force lost productive work time due to common pain conditions including headache, back pain, arthritis, and other musculoskeletal conditions. This lost productivity cost employers $61.2 billion per year, 77% of which was attributed to reduced performance while at work rather than work absence.

1.4   Course and Prognosis

Chronic pain is, by definition, persistent, and is expected in many cases to last indefinitely. It is usually not expected to completely resolve either with or without treatment. The goal of treatment, in most cases, is not to cure or "fix" the pain, as the underlying injury is either unknown or impossible to cure. Typically, the primary treatment goals are to reduce pain severity and improve function. Chronic pain and physical limitations can result in devastating changes in all areas of a person's life, and there are large individual differences in adjustment to these life changes. As the underlying source of the pain is usually not amenable to treatment, pain management and life adjustment are addressed in treatment instead.

Successful treatment can be defined by various outcome measures

The manner in which patients with chronic pain respond emotionally and behaviorally to pain varies considerably, depending on individual characteristics and external resources. Individuals with a broad repertoire of coping skills, flexibility of responses to adverse circumstances, and supportive family and friends may be able to make an adaptive adjustment to living with pain. For individuals with limited, passive, or rigid coping skills, or with inadequate social support, adjustment to living with pain is more likely to be poor and maladaptive.

Prognosis for successful treatment is influenced by temporal, individual, and environmental factors

Chronic pain taxes even the best coping resources; illness behaviors can develop and become increasingly ingrained, as do feelings of depression, apathy, and hopelessness. Consequently, the point at which treatment is initiated influences the course and outcome of pain management. A person seen early in the course of a pain condition may have a better response to treatment, or require less intensive treatment, than a patient who has been struggling with pain, depression, and deconditioning for many years. Without treatment, a number of factors can negatively influence the course and prognosis of adjustment to chronic pain. Among these factors are depression, catastrophizing, continued pursuit of a medical cure, and limited coping skills. However, each of these factors, when addressed within a cognitive-behavioral treatment paradigm, can show improvement and help facilitate adjustment.

As pain moves from acute to chronic, psychological factors play a greater role

1.5   Differential Diagnosis

Somatoform disorders are among the most common differential psychological diagnoses in the chronic pain population. The somatoform disorders include: somatization disorder, undifferentiated somatoform disorder, conversion disorder, pain disorder, hypochondriasis, body dysmorphic disorder, and somatoform disorder not otherwise specified. Too often, somatization, conversion, and hypochondriasis function as "catch-all" diagnoses that are made when pain and/or physical symptoms are of unknown etiology or when pain is considered to be "in excess of that expected." Patients may be referred to as "somatizers," even if they do not meet the DSM-IV diagnostic criteria for a somatization disorder. "Somatizing" may suggest that the patient is exquisitely attuned to even minor somatic symptoms, seeking attention or reassurance, or expressing emotional distress as physical complaints.

The somatoform diagnoses most often encountered in population are somatization and pain disorders. The diagnos matization disorder are quite stringent and require more tha pain of unknown etiology. This diagnosis usually requires an review, and the disorder may not become apparent until t relationship has been established over an extended period patient's full medical history unfolds.

The comparisons below are not meant to suggest that som never occurs in chronic pain populations. The caveat is that matization disorder, including lack of physical findings, may

Table 4
Comparison of Somatization Disorder and Chronic Pain

Somatization Disorder	Chronic Pain
Begins before the age of 30.	Can occur at any age.
Many physical complaints.	Not uncommon in older patients.
Treatment sought or significant impairment in social, occupational, or other important areas of functioning.	A history of multiple specialist visits and impairment in functioning are often seen.
Four pain symptoms.	Not uncommon in various pain disorders attributable to the disorder itself, e.g., arthritis, or to secondary pain areas resulting from guarding, or gait abnormalities.
Two gastrointestinal symptoms.	Common side effects of NSAIDs and other medications. [Symptoms resulting from medications are not considered as criteria for somatization disorder.]
One sexual symptom.	May result from the pain disorder, e.g., low back pain, abdominal pain, and/or adverse effects such as decreased libido and impotence associated with chronic opioid therapy. [Symptoms resulting from medications are not considered as criteria for somatization disorder.]
One pseudoneurological symptom.	Impaired balance can occur secondary to loss of sensation with a pain disorder such as peripheral neuropathy.
Not explainable by a known medical condition or substance (drug of abuse or medication).	See below.
If a medical condition is present, the complaints or impairment are in excess of what would be expected from history, physical, and lab findings.	Both peripheral and central sensitization can be found in chronic pain disorders due to facilitation of pain signal transmission from multiple sources. See Section 1.2.2.

a larger picture of chronic pain. It is important to be particularly careful in diagnosing somatization disorder in older patients, as multiple medical problems are not uncommon with aging. Two rules of thumb regarding the diagnosis of somatization disorder: (a) in most instances, avoid diagnosing somatization disorder solely on the basis of an initial evaluation because of the extensive medical history review usually required to make the diagnosis, and (b) unless the presence of somatization disorder can be established with certainty, it is better for the patient to include it only as a Rule out, since a diagnosis of somatization disorder can influence future medical treatment. The same cautions pertain to making a diagnosis of factitious disorder or malingering both of which entail the intentional production of pain symptoms for the purpose of assuming the sick role, obtaining financial compensation or drugs, avoidance of duties, criminal prosecution, or incarceration. However, it is important to recognize and diagnose somatization disorder when it is in fact present, as patients with this problem are often harmed by iatrogenic complications from unnecessary surgeries, invasive tests, and treatments.

> **Factitious disorder is the conscious production of physical symptoms to maintain the sick role**

The diagnosis of pain disorder encompasses three subtypes that differ in the degree to which the pain is thought to be initiated, maintained, or exacerbated by psychological factors. If psychological factors are considered to play a significant role in the initiation, severity, maintenance, or exacerbation of the pain complaint, the diagnosis of pain disorder with psychological factors (CPT code 307.80) may be made. If psychological factors are considered to play even a moderate role in the pain complaint, a diagnosis of pain disorder with psychological factors and a general medical condition may be made, and mental health CPT code 307.89 used. If psychological factors are thought to play a minimal or no role in the pain complaint, a diagnosis of pain disorder may be made, although this is not psychological diagnosis. The diagnosis of pain disorder is not appropriate if pain is better accounted for by a mood, anxiety, or psychotic disorder. To qualify for any of the three subtypes of pain disorder, the pain must cause impairment in functioning, and must not be intentionally produced as in malingering or factitious disorders.

> **Diagnosis of pain disorder includes three subtypes**

Pain disorder is a rather problematic diagnosis. Its definition evolved from a previous diagnostic category of psychogenic pain, and its very inclusion within the somatoform disorders implies a dichotomy between somatogenic and psychogenic pain. In addition, this diagnosis depends upon clinical judgment to determine when, and to what extent, psychological factors play a role in the overall picture of chronic pain.

> **Health and behavior codes are based on the presenting medical problem, not DSM-IV diagnoses**

However, as an appropriate use of pain disorder with psychological factors and a general medical condition, consider a person with severe arthritis who is no longer able to maintain many everyday household chores to which the family has responded in an angry and blaming manner. The patient's pain complaints increase, she becomes increasingly resentful, refusing to engage in any activities, and spending the day in bed with the door closed to avoid contact with her family. Although a clinician will have to decide whether, or to what extent, her pain is exacerbated by family dynamics, the diagnosis of pain disorder with psychological factors and a general medical condition would capture the problematic behaviors in this case, and point toward the appropriate treatment.

With the introduction of the health and behavior CPT codes (see Chapter 3), a diagnosis of the Axis III medical condition, e.g., chronic low back pain, may now be used as the primary diagnosis. The diagnosis and CPT code often more accurately reflect both the underlying physical problem for which the patient was referred and the focus of treatment.

1.6   Comorbidities

Individuals with chronic pain often have a wide range of physical and emotional problems, either as antecedent conditions or as consequences of the development of pain. These conditions can influence pain perception and adaptive coping. Some of the most common comorbidities in chronic pain are: sleep disorders, depression, anxiety disorders, and alcohol and substance abuse.

1.6.1   Sleep Disorders

Sleep disturbance is a significant problem among patients with chronic pain. Inadequate sleep can lead to a vicious cycle of fatigue, poor energy, and low motivation. This can, in turn, affect the patient's mood state, often by worsening depression and anxiety. Fatigue, poor motivation, anxiety, and low mood can influence pain perception and, continuing the cycle, further worsen sleep. Across studies with various chronic pain populations, the prevalence of self-reported sleep disturbance has ranged from 50% to 88%. The severity and characteristics of pain-related sleep disturbance, including subjective sleep quality, sleep latency, sleep duration, and daytime dysfunction, suggest that

Severe sleep disturbance is common

Table 5
Factors That Contribute to Sleep Disturbance

- Pain intensity

- Depression
  - Sleep disturbance may reflect depression. Sleep disturbance is a symptom of depression, and the prevalence of depression is high in the chronic pain population (Chui et al., 2005).

- Behavioral conditioning and poor sleep habits
  - Sleep may be so disturbed that patients often attempt to "make up" sleep with extended daytime naps or by sleeping late into the day.

- Medications (Onen, Onen, Courpron, & Dubray, 2005)
  - Aspirin and ibuprophen can increase sleep latency and awakenings, and decrease slow-wave sleep.
  - Opioids can decrease REM sleep, and increase sleep latency and night-time awakening.

- Arousal
  - Associated with pain.
  - Cognitive arousal including rumination, worry, depressive cognitions, and intrusive thoughts (Smith et al., 2000).

chronic pain patients report levels of sleep disturbance similar to those seen in primary insomnia (Smith, Perlis, Smith, Giles, & Carmody, 2000).

Sleep disturbances in pain patients are often treated with a low dose of an antidepressant such as amitripyline or trazodone. Patients should receive sleep hygiene education, as sleep can be disrupted not only by pain but also by a lack of temporal structure, maladaptive sleep behaviors, and other poor health habits. (See Chapter 4.)

Severe sleep disturbance is common

1.6.2   Depression

Depression is common in patients with chronic pain, as it is in patients with other chronic medical disorders. Epidemiological studies have attempted to document the prevalence of depression in the chronic pain population, as well as to determine whether a causal relationship exists between pain and depression.

Several factors make it difficult to obtain accurate estimates of the prevalence of depression in the chronic pain population. The first has to do with whether depression is defined as a mood state, a symptom, or a syndrome, and how it is measured. Prevalence estimates may vary depending on the definition of depression, and on whether mild depressive disorders such as dysthymia and adjustment disorder with depressed mood are included or excluded. Assessment methods range from self-report questionnaires to structured interviews with strict diagnostic criteria. The stringency of the criteria with which depression is diagnosed also affects prevalence estimates.

The second difficulty is that there are overlapping symptoms between chronic pain and depression. The DSM-IV criteria for major depression include a number of somatic symptoms such as insomnia, fatigue or loss of energy, changes in appetite and/or weight, and diminished ability to think or concentrate, all of which may be partially or entirely attributable to the pain itself or the medications used to treat it. The problem of overlapping symptoms also exists in other medical conditions. Some authorities have recommended modified diagnostic criteria for major depression in the chronic pain population in which the symptoms attributed to pain would be omitted or substituted with alternative symptoms. However, most attempts at changing the diagnostic criteria for depression in the chronic pain population have not improved the accuracy of diagnosis and have yielded a high rate of false negatives. Thus, the DSM-IV criteria are still recommended.

Some medications, such as cortico-steroids, can result in depressive symptoms

In the DSM-IV-TR (American Psychiatric Association, 2000), symptoms of depression include: feelings of sadness; loss of interest in usual activities (anhedonia); diminished ability to think or concentrate; excessive or inappropriate feelings of guilt; fatigue or loss of energy; sleep, appetite, and weight disturbances; psychomotor agitation or retardation; and thoughts of death or suicide or a suicide attempt. The symptoms must cause significant distress or impairment and must not be attributable to effects of medication, substances, or a general medical condition. Although the prevalence of depression in the population of patients with chronic pain has been estimated to be as low as 10% to as high as 100% (using self-report measures), more stringent criteria have placed the estimate at 30–54% (Banks & Kerns, 1996).

Low mood or anhedonia must be present for a diagnosis of depression

Medically ill patients often resist a diagnosis of depression

Pain and depression may be associated in several ways: (a) depression may be a consequence of coping with pain; (b) depression may precede the onset of chronic pain; and (c) pain and depression may co-occur. Persons with chronic pain suffer not only from pain, but also with physical limitations and multiple losses. Patients with chronic pain may be unable to maintain employment, which can lead to changes in economic status, loss of structured daily activity and changes in self-image and self-worth. Physical limitations often result in an inability to participate in sports and recreational activities, and even less physically demanding activities such as gardening, walking the dog, shopping, or self-care. For a variety of reasons, including fatigue, feeling "outside of things," and feeling misunderstood by others, people with chronic pain can become socially isolated and withdrawn from family and friends. Banks and Kerns (1996) present a diathesis-stress model of the association between pain and depression. They suggest that individuals bring to the experience of chronic pain certain vulnerabilities, or diatheses. These may include negative cognitive schemas, such as the tendency to make internal, stable, and global attributions for events, or deficits in coping skills. When the multiple stressors of chronic pain are experienced, these diatheses are activated. A negative or helpless view of life, feelings of lack of control, or inadequate coping resources, may produce a dysphoric mood or even trigger a full-blown major depressive episode.

"Masked depression" implied that a person presented with somatic, as opposed to emotional, symptoms

The "antecedent" hypothesis suggests that pain is a form of "masked depression," particularly in individuals with poor insight into their psychological functioning or limited ability to express their emotional states. It also suggests that individuals who express emotion in "the wrong channel," i.e., through physical complaints, are histrionic or alexythymic, and that their somatic focus serves as a defense against more threatening psychological emotions or conflicts. The concept of "masked depression" does not provide an adequate explanation of the relationship between pain and depression from the perspective of the biopsychosocial model. However, pain and depression do share neurochemical pathways, suggesting that a reciprocal interaction probably does exist. These pathways include serotonergic and noradrenergic neurotransmitters, and studying them may provide some insight into why depression might precede or co-occur with pain (Fishbain, Cutler, Rosomoff & Rosomoff, 1997).

Despite extensive attempts to identify a "pain-prone personality" research has borne out no such personality type

Depression in chronic pain patients is associated with nonadherence to treatment, greater pain intensity, poorer functioning, greater pain-related disability, and more use of passive coping (Fisher, Haythornthwaite, Heinberg, Clark, & Reed, 2001). Therefore, treatment is important no matter when depression occurs in the course of pain. Treatments include medications (primarily antidepressants) and nonpharmacologic interventions including various modalities of psychotherapy. Tricyclic antidepressants, e.g., amitriptyline and nortriptyline, and the newer serotonin norepinephrine reuptake inhibitors (SNRIs), e.g., duloxetine, have both antidepressant and analgesic properties. The selective serotonin reuptake inhibitors (SSRIs) are effective antidepressants with lower side effect profiles than the tricyclics, but are less effective analgesics.

Consider the side-effect profile before recommending an antidepressant

Suicidal ideation is common in the chronic pain population. Serious contemplation of suicide, and suicidal intent, increase with pain of longer duration and in those patients with depression. Completed suicides occur at 2–3 times the rate of those in the general population. However, the reported rates of suicide in the chronic pain population may be underestimated due to limited follow-up after discharge from pain clinics (Fishbain, Goldberg, Rosomoff, & Rosomoff, 1991).

1.6.3   Anxiety

Although the relationship between pain and depression is well researched and well accepted, McWilliams, Cox, and Enns (2003) found that the prevalence of anxiety disorders to be even higher than that of mood disorders in arthritis patients. They assessed mood disorders (depression and dysthmia) and anxiety disorders (generalized anxiety disorders, panic disorder, simple phobia, social phobia, agoraphobia with and without panic attacks, and posttraumatic stress disorder) with structured interviews. The estimated prevalences of mood and anxiety disorders in the clinical and general populations are presented in Table 6. Of particular relevance to understanding and treating chronic pain are pain-specific fear-avoidance beliefs, gender differences in the expression of anxiety, (Robinson, Dannecker, George, Otis, Atchsion, & Fillingim, 2005)

Pain-related fear avoidance is an anxiety-provoking thought that involves fear of movement

Fear of movement can become strengthened over time

Table 6
One-Year Prevalence of DSM-III-R Psychiatric Disorders

Diagnosis	Number of participants meeting diagnostic criteria (% in parentheses)		Inferential statistics	
	Chronic pain ($n = 382$)	General population ($n = 5495$)	x^2	p
Any mood disorder	83(21.7)	551(10.0)	32.16	<0.0001
Depression	77(20.2)	510(9.3)	26.53	<0.0001
Dysthymia	20(5.2)	128(2.3)	5.48	<0.01
Any anxiety disorder	134(35.1)	992(18.1)	21.54	<0.0001
Generalized anxiety disorder	28(7.3)	144(2.6)	9.10	<0.005
Panic disorder with or without agoraphobia	25(6.5)	103(1.9)	7.84	<0.01
Simple phobia	60(15.7)	456(8.3)	8.70	<0.01
Social phobia	45(11.8)	428(7.8)	5.91	<0.05
Agoraphobia with or without panic	32(8.4)	182(3.3)	6.52	<0.05
Posttraumatic stress disorder	41(10.7)	182(3.3)	16.29	<0.001

From McWilliams, Cox, and Enns (2003). Mood and anxiety disorder associated with chronic pain: An examination in a nationally representative sample. Page 129; reproduced with permission from IASP.

and the finding that multiple psychiatric diagnoses are associated with disability (McWilliams et al., 2003).

Generalized anxiety disorder (GAD) is characterized by excessive worry or apprehension lasting at least six months. The worry tends to focus on everyday activities (e.g., work, social, family). Generalized anxiety is associated with symptoms such as restlessness, fatigue, difficulty concentrating, irritability, muscle tension, and sleep disturbance. Individuals with GAD find it difficult to control their worry, and they report impairment in daily functioning because of excessive worrying. *Panic attacks* are characterized by discrete episodes of intense fear or discomfort associated with physical symptoms (palpitations; racing heartbeat; sweating; trembling or shaking; sensations of shortness of breath, smothering, or choking; chest pain or discomfort; nausea or abdominal distress; feeling dizzy, unsteady, or lightheaded; paresthesias; and chills or hot flushes) and affective symptoms (derealization or depersonalization, fear of losing control or going crazy, and fear of dying). *Posttraumatic stress disorder* occurs in response to a traumatic event such as experiencing, witnessing, or being confronted with an event that involves actual or threatened injury or death. In the chronic pain population, this diagnosis can be particularly pertinent for individuals whose pain was caused by a serious accident or injury. Symptoms of posttraumatic stress disorder include cognitive symptoms (intrusive thoughts or dreams about the event), affective symptoms (feelings of detachment or estrangement, diminished interest, restricted range of affect) and symptoms of increased arousal (difficulty with sleep, irritability, hypervigilance, and exaggerated startle response).

> **PTSD may result from assaults, disasters, or accidents any of which could result in chronic pain**

1.6.4   Substance Abuse

Individuals with a history of substance abuse are often found in medical settings and pain clinics because of accidents and injuries related to substance abuse, e.g., driving while intoxicated. Active substance abuse can seriously undermine effective pain management. Individuals with an active addiction may experience increased pain and/or sympathetic arousal, which occur with withdrawal from alcohol, cocaine, or other drugs, and which can exacerbate an underlying pain condition. They may engage in high-risk behaviors when intoxicated, thereby increasing the chances of worsening a painful condition, or they may be unable to comply with treatment recommendations (Savage, 2002).

It is possible for patients with chronic pain who have a past history of substance abuse to have their pain effectively managed with opioids, particularly if their use of opioids is closely monitored, expectations about opioid use are clearly established, and the patient is actively involved in a recovery program such as Alcoholics Anonymous. Patients who are actively addicted should be referred to a rehabilitation program, maintain participation in a recovery program, and have their opioid use monitored. Past and current substance use history (prescription medication, alcohol, and illicit drug use) should be obtained from patients for whom chronic opioid therapy is being considered and from individuals about whom questions arise concerning possible misuse of opioid analgesics.

> **History of substance abuse is not, of itself, a contraindication for treatment with opioids**

Addiction Versus Tolerance and Dependence

Opioids are a mainstay for the treatment of chronic pain, yet they have been controversial for decades. This controversy has been fueled by:

- Patient and physician fears about patient addiction.
- Physician fears of legal and regulatory reprisals.
  - Lawsuits for alleged over- and underprescribing of opioids.
  - Loss of license to practice.
- Illegal uses of opioids.
  - Recreational use.
  - Diversion (any nonprescribed use of opioids).
- Concern about worsening pain from long-term use of opioids (opioid tolerance-induced hyperalgesia).

Medicolegal terminology has evolved over the years. Drugs that were at one time referred to as narcotics are now called opioids in medical, as opposed to legal, usage. Opioids are morphine-like medications that relieve pain by binding to opioid receptors in the nervous system. Opioids include natural opiates (drugs with a chemical structure similar to morphine) as well as synthetic opioids and the endogenous opioids (endorphins).

The definitions of addiction, tolerance, dependence, and pseudoaddiction present special challenges and are addressed separately here to clarify their relationships to the use of pain medications, particularly opioid analgesics. Opioid addiction is relatively easy to identify in individuals who are not being treated for chronic pain, since there exists no other legitimate rationale for the sustained use of opioids. In contrast, the diagnosis of opioid addiction in a person being treated for pain can be exceedingly difficult. Concerns about addiction are prominent among both patients and providers. Consequently, it is imperative to utilize the correct terminology in order to diminish the potential

Table 7
Opiates and Opioids

Classification	Name	Brand Name
Natural opiates	Morphine	
	Codeine	
Semisynthetic opioids	Hydromorphone	Dilaudid
	Hydrocodone	Vicodin, Lortab, Norco (hydrocodone + acetaminophen)
	Oxycodone	Percocet, Tylox (oxycodone + acetaminophen OxyContin (slow-release formulation of oxycodone)
Synthetic opioids	Methadone	
	Meperidine	Demerol
	Fentanyl and sufentanil	
	Propoxyphene	Darvocet

for misunderstandings that can lead to the undertreatment of pain or to the overuse of potentially dangerous medications.

Long-term administration of opioids often produces both tolerance and physical dependence. Tolerance refers to a need for higher and higher doses of the opioid to achieve the same pain-relieving effect. If long-term opioid therapy is suddenly discontinued, patients who are physically dependent will manifest symptoms of withdrawal which may include: dysphoric mood, nausea or vomiting, muscle aches, tearing, runny nose, dilation of the pupils, sweating, diarrhea, yawning, fever, and insomnia. Withdrawal symptoms resolve over a few days and can be treated, when necessary, with small, tapering doses of opioids. Physical dependence should not be confused with addiction.

In DSM-IV-TR, substance dependence refers to what is commonly called addiction. Substance dependence refers to a cluster of physiological symptoms and cognitions as well as patterns of behavior, and not the physiological dependence mentioned above that occurs with long-term use of an opioid analgesic.

Table 8
DSM-IV-TR Criteria for Substance Dependence

A maladaptive pattern of substance use, leading to clinically significant impairment or distress, as manifested by three (or more) of the following, occurring at any time in the same twelve month period:

1. Tolerance, as defined by either of the following:
   (a) A need for markedly increased amounts of the substance to achieve intoxication or desired effect.
   (b) Markedly diminished effect with continued use of the same amount of substance.

2. Withdrawal, as manifested by either of the following:
   (a) The characteristic withdrawal syndrome for the substance.
   (b) The same (or a closely related) substance is taken to relieve, or avoid withdrawal symptoms.

3. The substance is often taken in larger amounts or over a longer period of time than was intended.

4. There is a persistent desire or unsuccessful efforts to cut down or control substance use.

5. A great deal of time is spent in activities necessary to obtain the substance (e.g., visiting multiple doctors or traveling long distances), use the substance (e.g., chain smoking), or recover from its effects.

6. Important social, occupational, or recreational activities are given up or reduced because of substance use.

7. The substance use is continued despite knowledge of having a persistent or recurrent physical or psychological problem that is likely to have been caused or exacerbated by the substance (e.g., current cocaine use despite recognition of cocaine-induced depression, or continued drinking despite recognition that an ulcer was made worse by alcohol consumption).

From the *Diagnostic and Statistical Manual – Text Revision*, 4th ed. (2000), Washington DC: American Psychiatric Association. Page 197, used with permission.

Tolerance and withdrawal symptoms (physiological dependence), as noted above, are not uncommon with the long-term use of opioids for management of pain. Therefore, many individuals prescribed opioid analgesics for pain readily meet two of the three criteria. The third criterion needed to establish a diagnosis of substance dependence by DSM-IV-TR definition is met if unsuccessful efforts have been made to cut down on use of the substance. Patients who attempt to cut down on opioids use may be unsuccessful due to physical dependence (development of withdrawal symptoms) or increased pain or both. However, such physical dependence and tolerance do not constitute addiction. They will almost inevitably occur when prescribed opioids are taken solely for the relief of pain and when taken over a prolonged period of time.

For patients taking opioids for management of pain, criteria that indicate "drug-seeking behaviors" (e.g., obtaining prescriptions from multiple doctors), are more likely to suggest addiction. However, even the presence of behaviors such as taking medications faster than prescribed, requests for increased dosage and other "drug seeking" behaviors may reflect nothing more than unrelieved pain. This is known as pseudoaddiction, as the behaviors often mimic addictive behaviors but resolve when pain is adequately treated. Addiction to opioids is uncommon among patients prescribed opioids for pain although the exact prevalence is not known. Data suggest that the prevalence of addiction to opioids among pain patients is similar to the rate in the general population, that is, 3–19% (Fishbain, Rosomoff, & Rosomoff, 1992).

Distinguish drug-seeking behaviors from pseudoaddiction

In attempting to clarify what addiction is and is not, the following definitions were developed by the Liaison Committee on Pain and Addiction in 2001. The Liaison Committee was composed of members from the American Academy of Pain Medicine, the American Pain Society and the American Society of Addiction Medicine.

Addiction is a maladaptive set of behaviors

Because opioid addiction is a life-threatening problem, and vulnerable individuals potentially abuse opioids, it is important to recognize signs of abuse and addiction. Patterns of use suggestive of addiction include: multiple requests for early refills, lost or stolen medications or prescriptions, forged prescriptions, obtaining prescription medications from nonmedical sources (street, Internet) and the use of multiple prescription providers.

Addiction is characterized by the "three C's" – impaired control, compulsive use, and craving

---

Table 9
Definitions of Dependence, Tolerance, and Addiction from the Liaison Committee on Pain and Addiction

Physical dependence is a state of adaptation that is manifested by a drug class specific withdrawal syndrome that can be produced by abrupt cessation, rapid dose reduction, decreasing blood level of the drug, or administration of an antagonist.

Tolerance is a state of adaptation in which exposure to a drug induces changes that result in a diminution of one or more of the drug's effects over time.

Addiction is a primary, chronic neurobiological disease with genetic, psychosocial, and environmental factors influencing its development and manifestations. It is characterized by behaviors that include one or more of the following: impaired control over drug use, compulsive use, continued use despite harm, and craving.

1.7   Diagnostic Procedures and Documentation

Because pain is subjective, there are no reliable and valid objective tests with which to measure it. Severity of pain is usually communicated by the patient to health care professionals in the form of a numerical rating (e.g., 0 to 10 scale with 0 representing *no pain* and 10 being the *worst pain imaginable*), a verbal rating (e.g., slightly unpleasant to very intolerable) or a set of pictures illustrating facial expressions ranging from happy and smiling to sad and crying. Pain rating scales are often used as treatment outcome measures but are rarely used as the sole measure of successful treatment. Particularly in multidisciplinary settings, treatment success is usually measured by some combination of the following criteria: decreased pain intensity, improved function, return to work, decreased use of pain medications, decreased healthcare utilization, and improvement in mood. Examples of measures of pain intensity, disability, and mood are listed in tables below. For further examples and comparisons of measures, see Turk and Melzack's *Handbook of Pain Assessment* (2nd edition, 2001), and the article by Von Korff, Jensen, and Karoly in the December 15, 2000, edition of *Spine*, an edition devoted to the topic of assessment and outcome measures for back pain. Measures may vary depending on the population being evaluated; for example, the picture scale may be more effective with children than verbal and numerical pain rating scales. A battery of measures that are reasonably quick, easy to use and score and that provide a broad range of information might include the Numerical Rating Scale, the Multidimensional Pain Inventory, and the Center for Epidemiological Studies-Depression (CES-D). This battery provides information about pain severity, depression, and the extent to which pain interferes with everyday activities and relationships.

Table 10
Measures of Pain Intensity

Scale	Description
Verbal Rating Scale (VRS)	A list of adjectives describing levels of pain intensity. The list should include words describing the extreme points of pain intensity *(no pain to extremely intense pain)* and the gradations of pain between the extremes (e.g., moderate, strong, very strong, etc.).
Visual Analog Scale (VAS)	A 10 cm line labeled at one end by the descriptor *no pain* and at the other end by the descriptor *pain as bad as it could be*. Patients mark a point along the line that represents the intensity of their pain.
Numerical Rating Scale (NRS)	NRS may be an 11-point scale (0–10) or a 101 point scale (0–100) with 0 representing *no pain* and 10 (or 100) representing *pain as bad as it could be*. The patient is asked to mark a number from 0 to 10 (or 0 to 100) that best represents their pain intensity.
Picture Scale (PS)	Drawings of a range of facial expressions representing people experiencing various levels of pain, from no pain (happy and smiling) to severe pain (sad and crying). Each picture has a number, from 0–7, which represents the pain intensity score.

Table 11
Measures of Function

Measure	Description
Sickness Impact Profile (SIP) (Bergner, Bobbitt, Carter, & Gilson, 1981)	A 136-item measure of functional disability. Everyday activities in 12 categories (sleep and rest, emotional behavior, body care and movement, home management, mobility, social interaction, ambulation, alertness behavior, communication, work, recreation and pastimes, and eating) are measured.
Roland-Morris Disability Questionnaire (RMDQ) (Roland & Morris, 1983)	A 24-item health status measure derived from the Sickness Impact Questionnaire. It is designed to assess functional limitations due to back pain in areas of physical activities, housework, mobility, dressing, getting help, appetite, irritability, and pain.
Oswestry Disability Index (ODI) (Fairbank, Couper, Davies, & O'Brien, 1980)	A 10-item instrument designed as a measure for assessment and outcome for patients with back pain. Functional areas assessed include pain intensity, personal care, lifting, walking, sitting, standing, sleeping, sex life, social life, and traveling.
SF-36 (Ware & Sherbourne, 1992)	The SF-36 is a 36-item instrument for measuring physical and mental quality of life from the patient's perspective. It assesses limitations in physical activities, usual role activities and social activities because of health problems. It includes measures of pain, general health perceptions, energy, and psychological distress.
Pain Disability Index (PDI) (Pollard, 1984)	A 7-item self-report measure designed to measure the degree to which pain interferes with daily functioning. Areas of functioning include family/home responsibilities, recreation, social activities, occupation, sexual behavior, self-care, and life-support activity.
Multidimensional Pain Inventory (MPI) (Kerns, Turk, & Rudy, 1985)	A 52-item, 12-scale inventory divided into three parts. Part III assesses the extent to which patients perceive their pain interferes with participation in the following activities: household chores, outdoor chores, activities away from home, and social activities. Part I also includes an assessment of pain interference with vocational, social/recreational, and family/marital functioning.
Work Status	− Employed at usual jobLight duty − Receiving short-term or long-term disability − Unemployed (due to injury/pain or other) − Homemaker − Student − Retired − Receiving Social Security disability

Table 12
Depression Measures

Instrument	Description
Center for Epidemiological Studies-Depression (CES-D) (Radloff, 1977)	A 20-item self-report measure designed to assess major depression. The items divide into four factors: depressive affect, somatic symptoms, positive affect and interpersonal relations.
Beck Depression Inventory (BDI-II) (Beck, Steer, & Brown, 1996)	The BDI-II is a 21-item self-report inventory designed to measure the presence of depression. Each item is designed to assess specific symptoms or attitudes consistent with the diagnosis of depression.
Structured Clinical Interview for DSM-III-R (SCID) (Spitzer, Williams, Gibbons, & First, 1992)	The SCID is a semistructured interview to be administered by a clinical used for making Axis I DSM diagnoses. The SCID can be used to assess the presence or absence of a diagnosis of depression for the current episode (past month) and for lifetime prevalence.
Depression Interview and Structured Hamilton (DISH) (Freedland et al., 2002)	The DISH is a semistructured interview used to assess the presence and severity of major and minor depression and dysthymia in medically ill patients. It can be administered by mental health clinicians and trained research assistants.

2

Theories and Models of the Disorder

2.1 Dualistic Models

From the 17th century until well into the 20th century, the disease or biomedical model dominated the understanding and treatment of pain. René Descartes proposed that pain results from stimulation of specific receptors by disease or injury, and that a one-to-one relationship exists between the degree of injury and the experience of pain. Psychological problems, such as depression and anxiety, might result from the experience of pain, but do not have a direct influence on it. According to this view, when pain resolves, depression and anxiety should also resolve.

With the rise of psychoanalytic theory in the late 19th and early 20th century, emotions, personality characteristics, and psychological conflicts began to be considered as factors that influence the expression of pain. Pain, particularly pain with no or limited physical findings, was often considered to result from a conversion of emotional conflict into somatic symptoms. The site of the pain might be symbolic of the underlying conflict; for example, abdominal, groin, or genital pain suggested an underlying sexual conflict. Pain was believed to be either somatogenic or psychogenic. If the intensity of pain and the level of disability were consistent with the degree of injury or other physical findings, the pain was considered to be somatogenic. Pain and disability without physical findings, pain that extended beyond the expected time for healing, and pain that was "out of proportion to that expected" was considered to be psychogenic.

Conversion disorder was considered to be a defense mechanism

2.2 Gate-Control Theory

In 1965, Ronald Melzack and Patrick Wall questioned the direct one-to-one relationship between intensity of stimulus and pain perception, and the dualistic concept of psychogenic versus somatogenic pain. They suggested that the intensity and quality of pain were determined by both physiological and psychological variables. Their gate-control model proposed that the transmission of pain-related nerve impulses is modulated by a "gating" mechanism at the dorsal horn of the spinal cord. This mechanism is influenced by the balance between large- and small-diameter nerve fiber activity, with small-diameter fibers facilitating transmission (i.e., opening the gate) and large-diameter fibers inhibiting transmission (closing the gate). It also proposed that processes in the brain modulate the gating mechanism that underlies the

The concept of a "gate" serves as a metaphor for understanding pain modulation

behavioral and experiential characteristics of pain. Although there have been substantial advances since 1965 in the understanding of the neurophysiology of pain transmission, the gate control model remains an important heuristic for understanding and treating pain.

Melzack and Casey suggested that the experience of pain is complex and multidimensional

In 1968, Melzack and Casey extended the gate-control model to better account for the motivational, affective, and cognitive aspects of pain. According to their extended model, sensory inputs are not the only determinants of pain. Pain is also determined by cognitive evaluations of its meaning, and by emotional responses that serve to motivate behavior. Thus, pain comprises not just one but three dimensions: a sensory-discriminative dimension, a cognitive-evaluative dimension, and an emotional-motivational dimension. Each of these three dimensions has a reciprocal influence on the others. Specific areas of the brain process information regarding the location, duration, and intensity of pain, while others process its unpleasantness. Central nervous system processes evaluate sensory input in the context of past experience, beliefs, and attributions.

The gate-control theory proposed that pain is modulated at the level of the spinal cord by both peripheral and central nervous system inputs. There are both facilitory and inhibitory factors that increase or decrease the degree of perceived pain. That is, they "open" or "close" the gate. The higher order factors that modulate the perception of pain include attention, mood, expectations, and beliefs. For example, attention directed away from pain closes the gate, whereas attention directed toward pain opens it. By recognizing that pain is influenced by multiple factors, the gate control model transformed the understanding of individual differences in the expression of pain and greatly expanded the range of potential interventions. Psychological processes were no longer seen as mere reactions to pain, but as primary mediators in the perception of pain.

2.3   Biopsychosocial Model

The biopsychosocial model is an interactive and dynamic model

Engel proposed the biopsychosocial model in 1977 and further developed it in the 1980s and 1990s. It emphasizes the dynamic interactions between biological, psychological, and social variables in chronic pain. The biological components include ascending and descending neural pathways and biochemical processes. The psychological components include attention, thoughts, emotions, expectations, beliefs, and attributions. The social aspects range from sociocultural expectations to interpersonal interactions, particularly within the family, that shape learned responses to pain. The interactions among these three components are continuous and reciprocal.

2.3.1   Operant Conditioning Model

In 1976, Wilbur Fordyce proposed a behavioral model of chronic pain based on Skinner's theories of operant conditioning. Fordyce was a pioneer in the behavioral treatment of chronic pain and was instrumental in establishing

Table 13
Premises Underlying the Operant or Behavioral Model

Acute injury	Chronic pain
Hurt versus harm	
Pain serves as a biological signal of harm. It informs the person to stop activity and seek care.	Less direct relationship between hurt and harm. Pain may no longer function as an important biological warning.
Cessation of activity	
Bed rest, care seeking, avoidance of usual activities and the use of analgesics is adaptive. These behaviors allow for healing. When healing is complete, pain resolves and normal activity resumes.	Bed rest, cessation of activity and exercise, avoidance of usual activities often leads to deconditoning and exacerbation of pain. Decreased activity becomes increasingly maladaptive.
Shift of contingencies	
Pain behaviors are maintained by nociceptive factors.	Social/environmental factors begin to play a greater role in pain behaviors. Increased attention and release from responsibility can positively reinforce pain behaviors. Lying or sitting down may negatively reinforce pain behaviors.

one of the first pain management centers in the country, at the University of Washington in Seattle. In the operant conditioning model, acute pain behaviors, although initiated by a traumatic injury or disease, are reinforced by interpersonal and environmental factors. Over time, with continued reinforcement, patients develop pain (or illness) behaviors. Fordyce proposed a behavioral treatment paradigm based on reducing the reinforcement of specific pain behaviors (e.g., rest or requests for medication) and positively reinforcing adaptive behaviors (e.g., resumption of normal daily activities).

Fordyce (1976) described pain behaviors that could be reinforced by interpersonal or environmental contingencies. There are both positive and negative reinforcers for pain behaviors. Positive reinforcement strengthens a behavior by providing pleasant or rewarding consequences for it, thereby increasing the likelihood that behavior will recur. Negative reinforcement strengthens a behavior by withdrawing an aversive or negative consequence. Behaviors that enable the individual to escape from or avoid an aversive stimulus tend to recur in its presence.

Treatment in the behavioral or operant paradigm focuses on modifying environmental contingencies to reduce disability and improve function. In the past, this form of behavioral treatment was often provided in an intensive inpatient program. Nowadays, it is more often provided on an outpatient basis. Behavioral treatment includes providing positive reinforcement for well behaviors such as those associated with increased activity and physical conditioning, and withdrawal of reinforcement for maladaptive pain behaviors. The patient's family is included in the treatment. Family members are taught about

In behavioral treatment settings, well-behaviors are positively reinforced

---

Table 14
Pain Behaviors and Reinforcement Contingencies

Verbal and observable pain behaviors:
- Groaning, moaning, sighing, limping, guarding.
- Requests for medication or assistance.

Negative reinforcement:
- Time spent sitting or lying down (avoidance of pain with standing or walking).
- Release from aversive activities and/or responsibilities.

Positive reinforcement:
- Attention from family, friends, health care providers.

Financial reinforcement:
- Injury-related litigation.
- Disability payments.

---

pain, reinforcement contingencies, well and illness behaviors, and ways to help the patient maintain treatment gains in his or her home environment.

"Exercising to success" is an example of changing behavioral contingencies to increase well behaviors. Prior to the development of operant conditioning programs, patients were generally advised to exercise to the point of experiencing pain, at which point they were instructed to rest. Because rest tends to relieve exercise-induced pain, this approach inadvertently reinforced any pain behaviors that occurred during exercise. In the behavioral treatment paradigm, patients are instead instructed to exercise for a specific (achievable) length of time or to a specific number of repetitions before resting. Consequently, rest reinforces the successful completion of exercise rather than the termination of exercise due to pain.

2.3.2   Cognitive-Behavioral Model

The cognitive-behavioral model built on the operant model. It integrates principles of operant treatment (e.g., changing contingencies of reinforcement, skill building, and the inclusion of families), with cognitive theory and therapy. A basic premise of cognitive theory is that perceptions of the world are filtered through personal history, beliefs, expectations, and attributions. Cognitions influence perception, emotions, and behavioral responses, including those involved in the experience of pain. This approach was initially developed by Aaron Beck in 1976 as a means of understanding and treating depression. While treating depressed patients, Beck noticed that patients perceived themselves and events negatively, often despite apparent successes and skills. He investigated whether changing a patient's negative cognitive filter could change his or her emotional responses, and found that this is indeed possible; depression responds to correction of distorted negative thinking. Cognitive therapy challenges distorted or dysfunctional cognitions and restructures them to improve the patient's self-image and to create a more adaptive view of his or her problems and circumstances. Cognitive therapy has been used as treat-

CBT requires active participation from the patient

ment for many other problems and disorders, including adaptation to chronic medical diseases, PTSD, alcohol dependence, anxiety, and pain.

Cognitive-behavior therapy is a collaborative effort, and requires active involvement from the patient and the therapist. The cognitive-behavioral model includes the patient as an active agent of change, in contrast to the operant conditioning model which views individuals as passively shaped by external reinforcement. In the chronic pain setting, this type of therapy often begins with education about chronic pain and the factors that modulate it. Negative cognitions that contribute to feelings of depression, helplessness, and lack of control are identified and restructured. Misperceptions, maladaptive beliefs, unrealistic expectations, fears, and negative assumptions are addressed. Treatment often includes developing techniques for redirecting attention away from pain, helping patients learn coping skills for managing pain, integrating coping skills into everyday life, and formulating plans for relapses.

2.3.3   Multidisciplinary Management

Psychological interventions for chronic pain have evolved along with the models discussed above. However, psychological therapies are rarely used as the sole treatment modality. Because of the complexity and multidimensionality of pain, single-modality treatments are not as effective as multimodal approaches. Psychological therapies are usually combined with medical treatments such as interventional pain procedures, medication management, and physical therapy.

Multidisciplinary treatment of pain originally developed from Dr. John Bonica's interactions with soldiers he treated while serving in the U.S. Army at Madigan Hospital during World War II. He found that while some patients responded to the existing treatments for pain, others did not. At the time, little was known about the treatment of chronic pain, and Bonica consulted with colleagues from other disciplines in an attempt to gain a better understanding of the complex experience of pain. This consultative process eventually developed into a multidisciplinary team approach in patients underwent a series of discipline-specific evaluations. The results of the evaluations were discussed at multidisciplinary team meetings. Bonica established multidisciplinary pain clinics in the 1940s and 1950s to serve the needs of soldiers injured during World War II. He established the multidisciplinary pain program at the University of Washington in Seattle in 1960 and pain management facilities proliferated rapidly during the1970s and 1980s.

Pain management facilities can be classified according to the type of patients seen for treatment and the variety of disciplines involved in evaluation and treatment. Disciplines that might be found in a multidisciplinary program include: anesthesiologists, neurologists, neurosurgeons, nurses, occupational therapists, pharmacists, physiatrists, physical therapists, and psychologists.

The First International Pain Meeting was held in Washington State in 1974

The International Association for the Study of Pain grew from the 1974 meeting

Table 15
Classification of Pain Centers and Clinics

Major Comprehensive Pain Center	Space and personnel devoted to evaluation and treatment of the multiple aspects of chronic pain. Includes a professional staff representing at least 5 disciplines with a full time support staff, organized evaluation and selection processes, therapies for a full range of problems, a training program, and systematic program evaluation.
Comprehensive Pain Center	Organized facility with personnel to evaluate and treat physical and psychosocial aspects of chronic pain.
Syndrome-Oriented Pain Center	Organized facility that offers treatment for a particular pain condition, e.g., low back pain clinics, headache clinics.
Modality-Oriented Pain Center	Offers therapy based on the clinic specialty, e.g., nerve block clinics, biofeedback clinics, acupuncture clinics.

3

Diagnosis and Treatment Indications

3.1   Referral Questions and Medical Record Review

This chapter will focus on assessment, diagnosis, and treatment planning for chronic pain patients who are referred for psychological evaluation. Some of the reasons why a patient might be referred for a psychological evaluation are listed in Table 16.

A careful review of the patient's medical records can provide information about the reason for referral, treatment history, and medication use. Because this can help focus the initial interview and treatment planning, it is advisable to request and review medical records from the referring physician prior to the initial psychological evaluation. The evaluation provides the foundation for diagnosis and treatment planning and, because pain is a complex problem, there are usually numerous issues to address. These may include: the patient's beliefs, expectations, and negative cognitions related to pain; symptoms of depression and anxiety; how well the patient and his or her family are adjusting to changes in family roles; comorbidities such as sleep disorders; and the patient's coping skills. An example of a questionnaire that may be used for an initial evaluation can be found in the Appendix.

Patients with chronic pain often resist referrals to mental health professionals. By the time they present for mental health services, many patients have already seen a number of physicians and other health care providers,

Discuss reasons for referral with the patient

Table 16
Reasons for Referral for Psychological Evaluation

- Assessment of psychiatric disorders.
- Evaluation of psychosocial factors that may be influencing coping, hindering treatment adherence, or affecting treatment effectiveness.
- Presurgical evaluation, e.g., for spinal surgery or neuroaugmentative procedures such as spinal cord stimulators or intrathecal drug delivery systems.
- Evaluation of substance use history and risk.
  - Candidacy for initiation of chronic opioids.
  - Potential for prescription medication misuse or abuse.
  - Questions concerning current abuse of alcohol or illicit drugs.
- Referral for psychological interventions targeting depression, anxiety, family issues.
- Referrals for psychological interventions for management of chronic pain.

> **Clinical Pearl**
> **Introduction to a Psychological Evaluation**
>
> "We know that people with chronic pain experience not only pain but also many changes in their lives. Pain can affect your ability to work, to be involved with sports and other activities you previously enjoyed, to go out with friends or play with your children. We know that people who experience chronic pain can have problems with their sleep, their moods, and their relationships with others. Your doctor asked you to meet with me so that we can get a better understanding of how pain is affecting your life. If I think that I can help you with any of the problems that the pain may be causing for you, we can talk about that toward the end of our meeting."

Patients are usually willing to discuss the impact of pain on their lives when they understand why they were referred

some of whom may have implied, or stated outright, that their pain is purely psychogenic. It can be challenging to establish a therapeutic alliance with patients who respond to a psychological referral with defensiveness, suspicion, or hostility. The introduction above can help assuage the patient's initial defensiveness.

Beginning the interview with a discussion of the patient's pain and its treatment to date focuses the session on the issues that most patients consider to be of primary importance. Obtaining a thorough medical history pertaining to pain treatment can provide clues to some important therapeutic issues such as the patient's expectations for treatment, anger about past treatments, and his or her understanding of the nature of the pain problem.

3.2   Guidelines for Assessing Medical History

3.2.1   History of Pain Complaint

Life changes can be as stressful as the pain itself

It is necessary to obtain a history of the patient's pain in order to understand subsequent psychosocial complications. The history should include questions about how long the patient has had pain, whether it was associated with an injury, and whether the injury was work- or accident-related. Responses to these questions may lead to an exploration of stressful circumstances such as unemployment, litigation, and financial problems. Asking about previous efforts to manage pain can help the clinician determine whether there is a pattern of "doctor shopping," and if so, whether this reflects uncontrolled or poorly controlled pain, an unrealistic hope for a medical cure, nonadherence to treatment recommendations, or problems with opioid abuse.

Ask about what the patient does for self-management of pain

Asking about diagnostic studies such as MRI, CT scan, and nerve conduction studies, can help to clarify your understanding of the patient's beliefs about the cause of his or her pain. Inquire about past and current treatments such as surgeries (how many and when?), interventional procedures, physical therapy, biofeedback, relaxation training, guided imagery, hypnosis, acupuncture, transcutaneous electrical nerve stimulation (TENS) units, chiropractic treatments, massage, and medications. A key question is whether any of these treatments provided any pain relief. If the patient states that "nothing helps," further questioning may clarify whether this reflects truly inadequate treatment or unrealistic expectations for a cure or complete pain relief. It is also possible that "nothing helps" because other complicating factors such as depression, fears, or secondary gain interfere with attempts to manage the patient's pain. Inquiring into the patient's expectations about treatment, such as whether he or she believes that a particular modality is likely to be helpful, can provide guidance for treatment recommendations, as these expectations can influence efficacy of treatment.

The initial evaluation should include questions about the patient's pain medications, such as the prescribed dosages and schedules of administration, and the extent to which the patient is adhering to the prescribed regimen. It should also include questions about whether these medications provide relief, whether they help the patient function better in everyday life, and whether there have been any adverse effects. If the reason for referral is related to the question of misuse of pain medications, consider asking the questions listed in the Clinical Pearl.

Even potent opioids reduce pain by only 30–40%

Clincal Pearl
Questions to Assess for Possible Misuse of Pain Medications

---

1. Are pain medications taken as prescribed?
   (A difficult distinction to make is whether the patient is misusing pain medications or overusing them because the dosage in inadequate to control pain [pseudoaddiction].)
   - If the patient has taken more medication than prescribed, under what circumstances does this happen?
   - How often does this happen?

2. Does the patient run out of pain medications early?
   - How often does this occur?
   - What does the patient do when a prescription for opioids runs out early?
   - Has running out early caused conflicts with a prescribing physician? More than once?

3. Who is prescribing pain medications?
   - A primary care physician or a pain management specialist?
   - Has the patient seen multiple pain specialists?
   - Has the patient been tried on various medications? Or were only one or two medications tried with minimal attempt to achieve a therapeutic dosage?

4. Has the patient ever obtained opioids from:
   - Friends or relatives?
   - The street or the Internet?
   - More than one physician?
   - Numerous trips to the emergency room?

5. Has the patient ever altered or forged a prescription?

6. Does the patient chew or 'shoot' long acting opioids?

7. Have the patient's pain medications (or prescriptions) been stolen or lost?
   (A difficult distinction to make is whether this indicates dangerous living circumstances or an attempt to disguise opioid misuse?)
   - How often has this occurred?

3.2.2   Pain Intensity, Location, Aggravating and Relieving Factors

Information about pain is provided by the patient's verbal report

Although pain intensity ratings are subjective, they are useful measures of treatment effectiveness. Inquiring about average, minimum, and maximum pain intensity can provide insight into how the patient understands and responds to pain. For example, when using a 0–10 rating scale, where 0 represents *no pain* and 10 indicates the *worst pain imaginable*, a patient might report that the pain is never less than a 10. This might suggest that factors such as hyperattentiveness to pain, or inability to distinguish fluctuations in physical sensations may be complicating pain perception. Patients may give high pain rating as a means of communicating their level of distress and frustration over inadequate pain relief.

Other characteristics of the patient's pain, such as its location and quality, should also be assessed. Some of the more commonly used measures of pain intensity, location, and quality are listed below.

Table 17
Pain Intensity, Quality, and Location Measures

Measure	Description
Visual Analog Scale (VAS) or Numerical Rating Scale (NRS)	Provides information about pain intensity. Quick and easy to use.
McGill Pain Questionnaire (MPQ) (Melzack, 1975)	Provides information about pain intensity, quality (sharp, burning, aching, etc.) and emotional responding. Has subscales for sensory and affective dimensions and a total pain score. Also available in a short form.
Pain Drawing	Provides information about location and quality of pain.

Inquire about aggravating and relieving factors by asking such questions as those in the Clinical Pearl.

Clinical Pearl
Questions to Determine Aggravating and Relieving Factors

What makes your pain worse?
- Is the patient overdoing certain activities, or not pacing everyday activities?
- Is the pain responsive to stressors?
- Does the pain limit physical intimacy and sexual activity, and does this affect personal relationships?

What makes your pain better?
- Does the patient use any self-management techniques to cope with pain?
- How does the patient perceive his or her role in the management of pain?
- Does the patient rely primarily on external resources for pain relief, e.g., pain medications?

3.2.3   Medical History

The patient's medical history can provide information about medical problems other than the chronic pain complaint with which a patient may be coping. Questions about surgeries, medical conditions, and medications should be included in the evaluation. The question of somatization disorder may arise if the patient has a complicated and extensive medical history. (See Chapter 1 for a more detailed discussion of somatization disorder.)

3.3   Guidelines for Assessing Cognitions

Experiences are filtered through individual beliefs, attributions, and expectations that are based in personal history and learning. Pain-related cognitions include beliefs about fairness, the personal meaning of the pain both for the present and the future, and expectations about appropriate treatment. Beliefs influence emotional responding, behavior (e.g., treatment seeking and interpersonal interactions), and adjustment to living with pain. Assessing the patient's beliefs about pain provides insight into his or her experience of, and response to, pain.

Assumptions and beliefs about justice, suffering, and fairness influence the pain experience

3.3.1 Beliefs and Expectations

With acute pain, healing of the injury and resolution of pain are treatment endpoints. With chronic pain, in contrast, management of symptoms, and development and maintenance of a meaningful and active lifestyle within optimized physical limitations, are the goals of treatment. If the patient believes that "the cause of my pain is being missed," or that an undiagnosed malignant disease underlies the pain, he or she will not be amenable to making the life adjustments that are necessary in order to cope with chronic pain. Before progress can be made toward helping the patient accept and adjust to pain, the question of what is causing the pain must therefore be resolved, or at least a reasonable explanation must be given and accepted. To elucidate the patient's understanding of the cause of his or her pain, consider asking the following questions.

Pain is influenced by individual beliefs and expectations about pain, illness, and treatment

---

Clinical Pearl
Questions to Pose to Determine the Understanding of the Cause of Pain

---

- How do you understand what is causing your pain?

- Has anyone given you a reasonable explanation of what is causing your pain?

- Do you feel as though something is being missed?

Active patient involvement is essential for treatment to be successful over the long run. The patient must practice and integrate ideas and insights gained from treatment into their everydays lives. Examples include maintaining a home exercise program, practicing relaxation exercises, pacing daily activities, and following sleep hygiene recommendations. If the patient is seeking a cure or complete relief from pain, most treatments will be perceived as failures. Chronic pain is, by definition, chronic. Asking such questions as: "When your pain is severe, what do you do?" "What are you hoping will be the outcome or the end goal of your pain management?" and "Of all the treatments you have tried so far, what helps the most?" will clarify the patient's beliefs about treatment and about the role that he or she expects to play in it.

Based on the patient's responses to these questions, it may be possible to provide an explanation for the patient's pain problem. In some cases, however, it is better to advise the patient to request an explanation from the treating physician. Even if there is no evident injury, pain can often be explained in etiological terms, e.g., as being due to tissue damage or neuropathy.

3.3.2　Cognition

In numerous studies of patients with chronic pain, cognitive distortions have been found to be associated with depression and poorer treatment outcomes. Catastrophizing, in particular, has been associated with greater pain intensity, emotional distress, and disability. Although there are numerous cognition distortions, examples of the more common ones are given below.

Because pain beliefs and cognitions span so many different dimensions, e.g., beliefs related to treatment, disability, control, etc., they can be difficult

Table 18
Common Cognitive Distortions

Catastrophizing	Magnifying the negative and anticipating the worst case scenario for events and experiences. Examples: "I can't stand this pain another minute!" "If my pain continues like this, I'll end up in a wheelchair."
Selective abstraction	Attending to negative aspects of experiences and disqualifying positive aspects. Examples: "So what if I managed to load the dishwasher today? I used to be able clean the whole house in a day." "If I can't keep up with my friends like I used to when we shop, then there's no point in going with them."
"Should" statements	Expectations (often unrealistic) about what one should or must be able to accomplish. Example: "I should be able to (clean the house, mow the lawn, dance) like I did before."
Overgeneralizing	Assuming that the outcome of one event inevitably applies to other or future events. Examples: "My pain always ruins my plans." "I'll never have a normal life again." "Nobody understands what I'm going through."

Table 19
Measures for Assessing Pain Beliefs, Cognitions, and Coping Strategies

Coping Strategies Questionnaire (CSQ), Rosensteil & Keefe (1983)
- Assesses six cognitive coping strategies (diverting attention, ignoring pain, reinterpreting pain, coping self-statements, praying or hoping, and catastrophizing).
- One behavioral strategy (increasing activity).
- Two self-efficacy items (perceived control over pain and ability to decrease pain).

Pain Catastrophizing Scale (PCS), Sullivan, Bishop, and Pivik (1995)
- Brief 13-item instrument.
- Examines three components of catastrophizing:
  – Rumination.
  – Magnification.
  – Helplessness.

Fear Avoidance Beliefs Questionnaire (FABQ), Waddell, Newton, Henderson, Somerville, and Main (1993)
- 16-item questionnaire; each item is rated on a 7-point Likert scale.
- Evaluates fear avoidance beliefs related to work and other activities.

to comprehensively assess during an initial interview. Questionnaires can help with the assessment of beliefs and coping strategies and examples are listed in Table 19. These measures could be used together in a battery as they assess different aspects of coping, beliefs, and cognitions. They are brief, self-report measures which may be completed prior to, during or following an interview. Particularly if the treatment approach is strongly cognitive, such a battery could provide excellent information about specific beliefs and cognitions on which treatment might focus. For a comprehensive review of pain assessment measures, see Turk and Melzack's *Handbook of Pain Assessment* (2nd edition, 2001).

3.4 Guidelines for Assessing Psychiatric Disorders

3.4.1 Behavioral Observations and Mental Status

Observations of the patient's behaviors and interactions during the initial interview should be documented. Record any observed pain behaviors, including actions that communicate the presence of pain, such as limping, guarding, moaning, groaning, wincing, grimacing, shifting or changing positions, or verbalizing pain. If pain behaviors are exceptional, it is useful to consider what is being communicated and why. Speech latencies, slurred speech, impaired attention or alertness, "nodding off," and difficulties maintaining a logical and goal-directed thought processes can suggest sedation or confusion due to medications or from other sources of cognitive impairment. If there is a question of cognitive impairment, consider using the Mini-Mental State Examination

36

(Folstein, Folstein, & McHugh, 1975) as a screening measure, and referring the patient for more extensive neuropsychological testing if necessary.

3.4.2   Depression

Depression can be underdiagnosed due to overlapping symptoms between pain and depression

As noted in Chapter 1, about 30–54% of patients seen in pain specialty clinics also suffer from depression. However, many patients are hesitant to talk about feelings of depression, for fear of having their pain complaints dismissed, or of being labeled as mentally ill. It is important to be sensitive to these fears. It can be helpful to approach the topic of depression as a normal response to pain-related losses and limitations.

The diagnostic problems associated with the overlapping symptoms of depression and other medical disorders have been noted, studied, and debated. Symptoms of depression, such as difficulties with sleep, memory, concentration, appetite, and libido, are also associated with chronic pain. Attempts have been made to modify the criteria for major depressive disorder, such as deleting the vegetative symptoms, substituting symptoms, or placing more emphasis on cognitive/affective symptoms, in order to reduce the risk of false positive diagnoses of major depression. However, these modifications do not increase the accuracy of the diagnosis of depression.

When evaluating depression, it is important to distinguish between depressed mood and major depressive disorder. To meet the criteria for a DSM-IV diagnosis of major depressive disorder, five symptoms must be present nearly every day for a period of at least two weeks and must cause significant impairment in social, occupational, or other areas of functioning. It is not uncommon for depressed chronic pain patients to be unaware of, or to deny, dysphoric mood. However, the DSM-IV criteria for major depression can be met even in the absence of dysphoric mood; *either* depressed mood *or* loss of interest or pleasure in usual activities (anhedonia) is required for a diagnosis of major depression. Loss of interest should be distinguished from inability to engage in previously enjoyed activities. Additional symptoms of major depressive disorder include: decreased (or increased) appetite with weight loss (or gain), insomnia or hypersomnia, psychomotor agitation or retardation, fatigue or loss of energy, feelings of worthlessness or excessive guilt, diminished ability to think or concentrate or indecisiveness, thoughts of death or suicide with or without a plan, or a suicide attempt. These symptoms should be assessed via a clinical interview, preferably supplemented with a self-report measure of the severity of depression such as the Beck Depression Inventory-II (BDI-II) or the Center for Epidemiological Studies-Depression (CES-D) Scale (see Table 12).

Fatigue, poor motivation, and hopelessness can negatively influence pain treatment

Sleep disturbance, which may be influenced by both depression and poorly controlled pain, can be assessed in conjunction with the evaluation for depression. A thorough evaluation of the patient's sleep patterns is essential, as inadequate sleep can influence his or her mood and ability to cope adaptively with pain.

When asked about suicidal ideation, chronic pain patients commonly report thoughts such as, "not wanting to go on like this," "wanting to get away," or "not wanting to wake up." Passive suicidal thoughts often communicate

Clinical Pearl
Questions to Determine a Patient's Sleep Pattern

- What time do you retire at night, and how long does it take you to fall asleep?
- Once asleep, do you stay asleep? If not, what wakes you up? Once awake, what do you do? Are you able to get back to sleep?
- What time do you get up in the morning? Do you feel rested? Do you stay up or go back to bed? Do you nap during the day? How long?
- Do you take any medications to help you with sleep?
- Do you use any techniques that help you sleep better?

the fatigue and sense of helplessness that can accompany intractable pain. These thoughts should be distinguished from feelings of profound despair and hopelessness that signal active suicidal ideation. Ask about suicidal intent, the presence of a plan, and the availability of means to carry out the plan. Assess risk factors such as family history of completed and attempted suicides, the patient's history of suicide attempts (and methods), and additional risk factors such as lack of social support, particularly in older patients. Suicide occurs in the chronic pain population at a higher rate than in the general population, so suicidal ideation should always be thoroughly assessed.

> The rate of completed suicides in the chronic pain population is probably underestimated

3.4.3   Anxiety Disorders

Subthreshold Anxiety Symptoms
Anxiety and worry do not, by themselves, necessarily constitute an anxiety disorder. However, pain-related anxiety can be relatively severe and can have clinical significance, even in the absence of a full-fledged anxiety disorder. Pain-related worries can include:
- Fears related to pain (fear of progressive or undiagnosed disease, fear of movement causing more damage).
- Fears about the future (fear of worsening pain, loss of mobility, long-term effects of medications, impact of pain and limitations on family and friends).
- Fears related to financial difficulties consequent to pain.

Panic Disorder
Panic disorder is accompanied by multiple physical symptoms that are often misinterpreted as potential threats to physical well-being. Patients with panic attacks often present to their physicians with cardiopulmonary complaints such as chest pain, rapid heartbeat, shortness of breath, sweating, and feelings of choking. They may also present with abdominal complaints such as nausea and abdominal upset, or with neurological complaints such as dizziness, faintness, trembling, shaking, and sweating. Panic attacks are subclassified with respect to whether they are accompanied by agoraphobia. Pain can limit a patient's ability or willingness to leave home, even in the absence of agoraphobia, so it is important to determine whether the patient becomes excessively fearful

when outside of the home. Ask socially isolated patients whether panic attacks contribute to their isolation.

Posttraumatic Stress Disorder

Pain may result from a traumatic event such as an accident. Almost one third of patients who experience an automobile accident requiring medical treatment meet the DSM-IV criteria for PTSD. Patients who have suffered physical or sexual abuse during childhood often meet the criteria for PTSD, and studies have noted histories of childhood sexual abuse in a high proportion of women reporting chronic pain. Posttraumatic stress disorder has been found in patients with a variety of other pain disorders as well, including atypical facial pain, fibromyalgia, and reflex sympathetic dystrophy.

3.4.4   Substance Abuse

Assessment of the risk for drug abuse and addiction is critical in the evaluation of patients being considered for treatment with chronic opioid analgesics. Unfortunately, none of the risk factors for addiction or misuse of opioids that have been identified are very strong predictors of patient behavior. However, if patients at risk for abuse or addiction can be identified, opioids can be carefully monitored until a pattern of adherence (or nonadherence) has been established. Patient and family histories of substance abuse, and history of legal problems, predict problematic behaviors such as claims of lost or stolen prescriptions, and the presence of illicit substances on urine toxicology screen (Michna et al., 2004). A study by Dunbar and Katz (1996) found that patients with a history of substance abuse who did *not* abuse opioid analgesics shared the following characteristics: The past history was significant only for alco-

---

Table 20
Evaluation of Alcohol and Illicit Drug History

- Past and current substance use history.
- Family history of substance abuse.
- Frequency of consumption.
- Amount consumed and over what period of time (daily, weekends).
- Age at which use of substances began.
- History of legal problems (incarceration, DWIs, or DUIs) related to substance use.
- Types of recovery programs, how often attended, and time frame for abstinence.
  - Attendance at AA or NA.
- Current social support.
- Signs of intoxication or withdrawal:
  - Sedation, cognitive changes, constricted pupils.
  - Sweating, flushing, rapid heart rate, dilated pupils.

hol abuse (or if there was history of polysubstance abuse, it was remote); the patient was attending a recovery program such as Alcoholics Anonymous; and the patient had good social support.

3.5   Guidelines for Assessing Daily Activity Patterns

Improving patients' ability to engage in normal daily activities is a primary goal of psychological interventions for chronic pain. Consequently, it is important to assess the patient's pattern of daily activities. What activities provide meaning and stimulation for the patient, and how is his or her day structured? How has pain affected his or her relationships with friends and family? What impact have pain, limitations, and losses of meaningful activities had on the patient's self-image and sense of self-worth?

3.5.1   Work and Everyday Activities

Many individuals with chronic pain stop working because of the physical demands of their job, fatigue, or the effect of medications. If the patient is not working, ask about the circumstances under which employment was discontinued.

The literature is mixed regarding the impact of Workers' Compensation and litigation on treatment

These factors can contribute to a loss (or lessening) of wages, anger about job loss, and stresses associated with the legal or workers compensation systems. If the patient is still working, address whether the pain affects his or her job performance, whether the job is physically demanding, and if any accommodations have been made.

It is not uncommon to find chronic pain patients who, over time, fall into a pattern of extremely limited daytime activity. Patients' activities can be limited to watching TV, sitting at a computer monitor, or dozing. The inability to engage in previously enjoyed activities, the sedating effects of medications, and the pain relief often experienced with sitting or laying down, can yield a sedentary lifestyle with little structure or meaning. This, in turn, can contribute to depression, fatigue, difficulties with sleep, physical deconditioning, limited endurance, and worsened disability.

Clinical Pearl
Questions to Determine the Impact of Pain on Work and Everyday Activities

- Did you leave work because you were unable to meet job demands due to pain?
- Did your pain result from a work-related injury?
- How did your boss and coworkers respond to your injury?
- Were you terminated from your job?
- Are litigation, workers' compensation, and/or disability payments involved?

It is informative to inquire about how the patient spends an average day, including everyday tasks such as household chores, yard work, or shopping. Does the patient engage in any pleasurable activities, such as going to movies or out to dinner, pursuing hobbies, or seeing friends? Does the patient gets up and dressed every day? How many hours are spent lying or sitting down, and how many hours are spent watching TV?

3.5.2   Relationships – Family and Friends

A good social support system positively influences how patients cope with pain

Chronic pain and physical limitations can affect a patient's marriage and influence his or her relationships with children, friends, and coworkers. Conversely, how the individual copes with pain can be influenced by the support, or lack of support, received from others. A spouse may become angry and resentful about having to return to work or take on a larger share of the household responsibilities. Family members may perceive the patient as "lazy" and as attempting to avoid responsibilities. Alternately, family members may become overly solicitous, anticipating the patient's every need and taking over the responsibility for his or her daily life. Under these circumstances, the patient is left with no active role in the family and can come to feel worthless. Patients can become socially isolated, rarely going out of the house. They may perceive themselves as unable to commit to invitations from friends, as pain too often dictates their ability to keep an engagement. The following questions can help to clarify how pain is influencing the patient's social interactions.

Clinical Pearl
Questions to Determine the Influence of Pain on Social Interactions

- How have pain and physical limitations affected your relationship with your spouse? How does he [or she] respond when you talk about pain?

- Has your pain affected your relationship with your children? In what ways?

- How have your friends responded? Do you go out with friends? Return phone calls? Accept invitations?

- Do you have any other sources of support such as from siblings, friends, your place of worship, or other organizations?

3.6   Additional Areas for Assessment

3.6.1   Anger

Although anger is not a psychiatric disorder, problematic forms of it are often seen in patients with chronic pain. Patients with chronic pain have often been involved in the medical system for years. They have seen many physicians, been referred for numerous treatments, and prescribed multiple medications. They may have been discharged by treating physicians despite continuing to suffer with pain, and bounced from one specialist to another. They may have received a host of conflicting or confusing diagnoses, and been subjected to implied or outright accusations of drug seeking, malingering or "somatizing." Patients are often involved in litigation over injury or disability, may be struggling with compensation or medical coverage issues with their workers' compensation carrier or become overwhelmed by complex medical insurance regulations. Consequently, patients with chronic pain are often very angry and frustrated. The patient's anger and the reasons behind it should be carefully assessed, as seeking a resolution for anger may be the primary focus of therapy.

3.6.2   Social History

Discussion of a patient's early history can provide important clues into his or her current responses to pain. It is useful to know whether the patient was raised around others with chronic pain or illness. If so, how did they cope with it? Was there physical, sexual, or emotional abuse in the household that either involved the patient directly or that he or she witnessed? Did the patient have strong, supportive relationships with parents and siblings, or was there discord and estrangement? Was there a history of psychiatric disorders, alcohol or drug abuse in the patient's family of origin? It is also helpful to assess similar issues in the patient's current relationships. If dysfunction in these relationships is longstanding, and if these problems preceded the onset of chronic pain, consider a referral to a family or marriage counselor. If the family or marital discord is primarily due to pain-related difficulties, these issues can often be addressed within the context of pain care.

> A personal history can provide important insight into how patients cope with adversity

3.6.3   Educational and Employment History

Information about the patient's educational and employment history is needed for treatment planning particularly if job retraining will be considered.

If the patient is interested in returning to employment but will need retraining to do so, consider a referral to a state-supported, or private, vocational rehabilitation agency.

> Social Security's "Ticket to Work" program helps people retrain and return to work

---

Clinical Pearl
Questions About Educational and Employment History

- Does the patient have a history of achievement in education, athletics, arts, or in his or her profession?

- Does he or she have a stable work history?

- Is his or her work physically demanding, and if so, is the patient struggling to meet these demands?

- Has the patient considered continuing in, or returning to, his or her previous employment, or retraining in a different field?

- What is the patient's current financial situation, and how has pain affected his or her financial well-being?

Table 21
Additional Assessment Measures

Measure	Description
Sickness Impact Profile (SIP) (Bergner et al., 1981) or SIP-68 (short-form) (DeBruin, Diederiks, DeWitte, Stevens, & Philipsen, 1994)	Measure of functional disability on 12 dimensions. Three combined dimensions of physical disability, psychosocial disability, and total disability.
West Haven-Yale Multidimensional Pain Inventory (MPI) (Kerns et al., 1985)	56-item measure with three sections. Section 1 assesses pain interference in various life domains; Section 2 assesses spouse and others' responses to patients pain; and Section 3 assesses activity involvement.
Patient Diaries	Daily event diaries can be used to assess pain, mood, sleep, uptime/downtime, socializing, medication use, use of pain management techniques.
Pain Anxiety Symptom Scale-20 (PASS-20) (McCracken & Dhinga, 2002)	Assesses pain-related anxiety. Composed of 20 items that assess the frequency with which an individual engages in certain thoughts or actions.

3.6.4   Presurgical Screening

The purpose of a presurgical psychological screening is to assess the patient's readiness for surgery, e.g., for spinal surgery or for implantation of neuro-modulatory devices such as spinal cord stimulators or intrathecal drug delivery systems. The following psychiatric diagnoses and psychosocial factors are contraindications for implantable devices and elective surgeries:

- Active psychosis.
- Depression with suicidal ideation.
- Current substance abuse.
- Current physical or sexual abuse.
- Inability to understand the functioning of a spinal cord stimulator or intrathecal device due to dementia, intellectual deficits, or psychosis.
- Inability to participate in perioperative care and rehabilitation.

If any of these factors are present, make recommendations for treatment, e.g., psychiatric evaluation for psychosis or severe depression, substance abuse treatment, protective services and counseling for abuse. Reevaluate following treatment. Patients may become candidates for implantable devices following resolution of these problems. Patients with dementia or severe intellectual deficits may become candidates for an implantable device if they have adequate assistance with daily living.

The following factors of themselves do not contraindicate surgery. However, as the number of risk factors present increases, the prognosis for a positive surgical outcome decreases.

- Current litigation or worker's compensation.
- Job dissatisfaction.
- Inadequate social support.
- Marital discord.
- History of abuse (physical or sexual).

Consider using the MMPI-2 (Hathaway et al., 1989), or similar psychological tests, as part of the presurgical evaluation. Such tests may shed light on the patient's attitude, coping style, and personality characteristics. Care must be taken in the interpretation of the MMPI clinical scales, particularly Scales 1 and 3, which contain somatic items and may be overinterpreted in the chronic pain population due to physical illness.

For a comprehensive explanation of presurgical assessment, see Andrew Block's book *Presurgical Psychological Screening in Chronic Pain Syndromes: A Guide for the Behavioral Health Practitioner* (1996).

3.7 Diagnosis and Treatment Recommendations

3.7.1 Diagnosis

Axis I psychiatric diagnoses will include clinical syndromes based on DSM-IV-TR classification such as major depression, adjustment disorders, substance dependence, etc. A diagnosis that is often made in the context of chronic pain, but which is a source of controversy, is Pain Disorder with Psychological Factors and a General Medical Condition (307.89). Part of the controversy centers on its classification as a somatoform disorder in the DSM-IV, which suggests a distinction between somatogenic and psychogenic pain. Nevertheless, the diagnosis of Pain Disorder with Psychological Factors and a General Medical Condition can be appropriate under certain circumstances. For example, it would apply to a patient with osteoarthritis of the neck and shoulder who is employed at a highly stressful job and whose pain worsens as job demands and deadlines increase.

Both the DSM-IV-TR and *International Classification of Diseases*, 10th revision (ICD-10; World Health Organization, 1992) systems for classification of mental disorders separate mental from physical complaints. The pain-related diagnostic categories in these systems are unfortunately based on an outdated dualistic model in which pain is considered to be either somatogenic or psychogenic.

The referring physician's ICD-10 diagnosis of the patient's pain became particularly relevant for providers of psychological services with the introduction of the health and behavior codes. Current Procedural Terminology (CPT; American Medical Association, 2007) is a system of terminology used to report medical procedures and services under public and private health insurance programs. The health and behavior CPT codes address the interface between medical conditions and psychological treatments. The health and behavior codes can be used in the absence of a mental health diagnosis and, even if an Axis I diagnosis is present, often reflect a more medical focus of treatment. These codes are billed in 15-minute increments, and may be used for evalua-

Table 22
Health and Behavior Assessment and Intervention Reimbursement Codes under the Current Procedural Terminology (CPT) Coding System

96150	Initial health and behavior assessment.
96151	Reassessment of a previously evaluated patient to determine the need for further treatment.
96152	Individual intervention sessions.
96153	Group intervention sessions.
96154	Intervention session with family and patient present.
96155	Intervention session with family of patient (patient not present).

tion, assessment, or treatment (group, individual, and family). Medicare, and many (but not all) private insurers, reimburse for health and behavior codes. More information about health and behavior codes is available at http://www.apa.org/practice/cpt_faq.html.

3.7.2   Treatment Plan

The goals of the initial psychological evaluation are: (a) to determine factors that may be influencing pain perception and coping and/or limiting attempts at rehabilitation, (b) develop a treatment plan that addresses these various factors, and (c) develop goals that could lead to specific treatment outcomes. By the end of the evaluation, it should be possible to formulate a treatment plan including, but not limited to, some of the following areas:

- Developing pain management techniques (relaxation, imagery, meditation).
- Developing pain coping skills (pacing activities, communication skills).
- Addressing dysfunctional and negative cognitions.
- Family sessions to address their adjustment to the patient's pain and limitations.
- Developing goals and meaningful daily activities.
- Improving socialization and social support.

3.7.3   Referrals to Additional Providers and Communication with Referring Physicians

Consider referring a patient when:

- You diagnose major depression, an anxiety disorder, or bipolar disorder, and psychotropic medication is appropriate. Consult with the referring physician, and consider referral to a psychiatrist.
- The patient is currently abusing alcohol or illegal substances. Refer for substance abuse treatment. If the patient is abusing prescribed opioids, consult with the prescribing physician.

- Marital (or family) stress is disrupting family life, and these issues preceded the patient's pain problem, consider referral for marital or family therapy.
- A patient who is not currently working and cannot return to his or her previous profession appears motivated to return to some type of work. Consider referral to a state or private vocational training agency.
- A patient is a candidate for a treatment that requires specialized psychological expertise, e.g., hypnosis or biofeedback. Refer to an experienced provider.
- The patient has no regular exercise program and has had little or no physical therapy. Refer to a well-trained physical therapist who is knowledgeable about working with patients with chronic pain. (Orders from a physician are required for physical therapy.)
- The patient's pain and related problems seem too difficult and complex. Consider referring him or her to a multidisciplinary pain management program (generally found within tertiary care hospitals).

It is advisable to send a copy or summary of the initial evaluation, as well as regular updates during the course of psychological intervention, to the referring physician. Because of the complexity of chronic pain, it is essential to maintain contact with the referring physician.

4

Treatment

4.1 Introduction

Pain is the most common symptom of medical illness and one of the most frequent reasons why patients seek medical care. Consequently, medical treatments for pain are among the most commonly prescribed therapies. There has been a tremendous growth in access to pain therapies over the past 20 years, and pain medicine specialists are now available at the vast majority of U.S. hospitals. During this same time, there have been remarkable advances in our understanding of the pathophysiology of pain. Despite these promising developments, pain is still undertreated, and pain treatments are often inadequate.

Pain is too often undertreated

Although many disease-related, individual, societal, and environmental factors influence pain and its management, a few realities broadly limit the provision of effective treatment for pain. These include the basic neurobiology of pain, the complexity of human pain (illness) behavior, and the high cost of pain therapy.

- Laboratory studies have shown that there are numerous, overlapping mechanisms for the detection, transmission, and modulation of pain signals, resulting in a pain signaling system that is redundant and robust. Although an analgesic may limit some portion of a particular pain signaling pathway, pain signals may be transmitted or modulated through other mechanisms. As more is learned about the complexity of pain signaling, it seems increasingly unlikely that the ideal analgesic (i.e., one that is sufficiently potent to control intense pain, that has limited adverse effects, is easy to administer, and is suitable for chronic administration) will ever be identified.

- Pain is expressed in a wide range of behaviors (e.g., crying out, limping, requesting assistance, filing for disability). In mature adults, pain behaviors are often very well practiced and resistant to change, even when appropriate therapies are available and utilized.

- Therapy for chronic pain is expensive. Newer medications often cost hundreds of dollars per month, and optimal management of pain may require more than one medication as well as extensive physical, occupational, cognitive-behavioral, and vocational therapies. Repeated surgical, or other palliative interventions may cost tens of thousands of dollars. In view of increasing limitations on health care expenditures, it is no wonder that optimal pain therapy remains out of reach for many patients, even within developed countries.

Although clinical pain management is not a simple undertaking, the humanitarian mandate to provide relief of pain is obvious, and effective therapies are available. Directly treating the pain-producing illness or injury should be the principle focus of treatment when feasible, since this may produce the most satisfactory pain relief. Even when treatment of the underlying illness/injury seems likely to be successful, concomitant use of pain relieving therapies, together with disease treatments, is generally appropriate and often necessary. With chronic pain, it is often the case that either direct treatment of the underlying problem is not possible or that even optimized treatments may fail to provide complete relief. Sometimes, treatments for the primary disease (surgery, radiation therapy, chemotherapy) may result in new or worsened pain. Because analgesic therapies often prove inadequate for the control of chronic pain, treatment must extend beyond efforts to reduce pain intensity. Chronic pain is a complex, multifactorial experience, so pain management therapies should be multidimensional or multidisciplinary. In general, chronic pain therapies strive to help the patient better manage pain and related symptoms, while maintaining or developing a meaningful and active lifestyle within optimized physical limitations.

> **Treatment of an underlying disease may not be possible or may not completely relieve pain**

When reasonable diagnostic investigations and appropriate primary disease treatments have failed to adequately resolve pain, it is necessary to focus directly on management of chronic pain. Persisting in futile efforts to diagnose and treat a suspected primary disease process can have unintended, adverse effects. Such efforts can:

- Subject the patient to increasingly invasive diagnostic or treatment procedures that pose a risk of iatrogenic complications.
- Add to patient frustration and lack of interest in or commitment to subsequent attempts at pain management.
- Delay patient access to appropriate management therapies and thereby contribute to physical deterioration and deconditioning.
- Divert resources of time, effort and money away from more useful management strategies.

4.2   Methods of Treatment

If optimized, disease-curative treatments have failed to resolve chronic pain, management strategies may include analgesic medications, behavioral or psychological therapies, physical therapies, injections, interventional procedures, and (rarely) other palliative procedures. These therapies often have both primary and secondary goals, and multiple disciplines can have overlapping treatment goals. For example, analgesics alleviate pain but also may improve pain-induced insomnia and consequently improve mood and energy. Conversely, antidepressants might alleviate depression and insomnia, with consequently improved tolerance to existing pain. Physical therapy might address specific muscle weakness contributing to pain, but might also include conditioning exercises to improve stamina and overall function. Psychological therapies focus on managing the consequences of pain and developing pain coping strategies, with which patients may experience pain of lessened intensity and a greater sense of control.

> **Improvement in one area of the pain cycle may result in improvement in other areas**

4.2.1   Medical Treatments

There is a wide range of medical treatments for chronic pain, with analgesic medications being the most commonly utilized. It is now well recognized, however, that the currently available analgesics have significant limitations in chronic pain management, including incomplete pain relief (especially with severe pain), adverse effects, and tolerance. There have been tremendous advances in our understanding of neurophysiology of chronic pain but, so far, they have not been translated into new analgesic therapies. The principal analgesics in clinical use today are the same ones that have been in use over the past two to four decades, or even longer. Fortunately, a wide range of medical therapies are available for chronic pain, including a large variety of analgesic medications. Although a detailed description of the clinical use of all of these therapies is beyond the scope of this text, some familiarity with available pain therapies is desirable so that multidisciplinary care can be well-coordinated and optimized. Further details are available in standard pain texts (Cousins & Bridenbaugh, 1998; Loeser, 2001; McMahon & Koltzenburg, 2006).

Analgesic Medications

Pain medications should be considered after weighing benefits against potential risks

The diverse array of medications with pain relieving effects are generally categorized as nonopioid analgesics (acetaminophen, nonsteroidal anti-inflammatory drugs), opioid analgesics (morphine-like agents), or adjuvant analgesics (anticonvulsants, antidepressants). In general, opioid is the preferred name for all analgesics that have a mechanism of action similar to morphine. Opiates are that subset of opioids that are derived from opium and/or have a chemical structure similar to morphine. In the past, opioid analgesics have been called narcotic analgesics, but "narcotic" is a pharmacologically imprecise term which is best used to designate potentially abusable, controlled drugs.

In most clinical settings, analgesic agents are used empirically. In other words, even the best available research findings do not necessarily provide clinicians with sufficient guidance as to what will or will not work in any given case. Consequently, a trial and error approach is often needed to find the optimal treatment for an individual patient. In addition, there are some areas of pain management in which there is little evidence to support commonly used therapies. The long-term use of opioid analgesics for the management of chronic, noncancer pain is a notable example. The use of any kind of medical therapy must be based on careful consideration of the potential benefits and risks. Because analgesics reduce pain intensity only temporarily, and generally do not contribute to the long-term resolution of pain, they must be used cautiously in order to avoid adverse effects.

Nonopioid analgesics include acetaminophen, aspirin along with other salicylates, and nonsteroidal anti-inflammatory drugs (NSAIDs). These agents are widely used in the management of acute and chronic pain of mild to moderate severity. Several are available without prescription, including aspirin, acetaminophen, ibuprofen, naproxen, and ketoprofen. These agents have limited efficacy, even at maximal therapeutic doses. While reasonably safe for most individuals, all of the nonopioid analgesics have potential toxicities that can limit their utility.

Table 23
Nonopioid Analgesics for Chronic Pain

Generic Drug (Trade Name)	Usual, single oral dose (mg/dose)	Maximum daily dose (mg/day)
Acetaminophen (Tylenol)	650–1000	4000
Aspirin	650–1000	5000
Nonsteroidal anti-inflammatory drugs (NSAIDS)		
Ibuprofen (Advil, Motrin)	200–800	3200
Celecoxib (Celebrex)	100–200	800
Diclofenac (Voltaren, Cataflam)	50	225
Etodolac (Lodine)	200–300	1200
Ketoprofen (Orudis)	50–75	300
Ketorolac (Toradol) Risk of peptic ulceration limits use to 5 days. Contraindicated in hepatic disease	10	40
Meloxicam (Mobic)	7.5–15	7.5–15
Nabumetone (Relafen)	500–750	2000
Naproxen (Aleve, Naprosyn)	220–500	1500
Oxaprozin (Daypro)	600	1800
Piroxicam (Feldene)	10–20	20

Acetaminophen is a modestly effective analgesic that appears to dampen pain signal transmission in the central nervous system. In typical doses, it is generally safe and well tolerated. It is recommended as the first line analgesic or antipyretic for infants, children, and also for adults at increased risk for peptic ulceration. However, excessive doses of acetaminophen, or even therapeutic doses in individuals with chronic alcohol use or liver disease, may result in potentially fatal hepatotoxicity.

Aspirin (acetylsalicylic acid) has been in clinical use since 1899 and remains a widely utilized analgesic and antipyretic. The efficacy of aspirin in management of acute pain has been well documented in randomized, controlled trials (RCTs). For chronic pain, aspirin and other salicylates appear to have similar analgesic potency as NSAIDs. Gastrointestinal toxicity (gastritis, bleeding, and peptic ulceration) are more common with aspirin than with other nonacetylated salicylates (salsalate, choline salicylates) and NSAIDs. Due to increased risk of gastrointestinal bleeding, chronic alcohol use is a relative contraindication to chronic use of aspirin. Due to risk of worsening renal function, aspirin should also be avoided in patients with renal insufficiency. Based on RCTs, NSAIDs appear to be more efficacious than acetaminophen in controlling pain due to osteoarthritis and rheumatoid arthritis. Gastrointestinal toxicity (gastritis, bleeding, peptic ulceration) is the most common adverse effect limiting clinical use of NSAIDs. Due to risk of worsening renal function, NSAIDs are contraindicated in individuals with renal insufficiency.

Nonopioid analgesics can have adverse side-effects

Opioid analgesics include all agents which have an analgesic effect similar to that of morphine, acting through specific opioid receptors in the peripheral and central nervous systems. Opioid analgesics include naturally-occurring agents derived from opium (morphine, codeine), chemically manufactured agents (e.g., hydromorphone, fentanyl, methadone), and the body's own endogenously-produced endorphins. Although the analgesic effect of opium has been known for over 2000 years, opioids are still the most potent and most widely applicable analgesics available today.

Although extensively used in clinical practice for control of both acute and chronic pain, there is relatively little clinical research data regarding the long-term use of opioid analgesics in chronic pain. Most of the available evidence supporting the use of opioids for chronic pain comes from uncontrolled clinical case series, with follow-up periods of up to a year or two. A few RCTs of up to six to eight weeks duration have demonstrated efficacy of opioids in chronic

Table 24
Opioid Analgesics for Chronic Pain, with Estimates of Equivalent Doses Used at the Washington University Pain Management Center

Generic name (Trade name)	Elimination (t½) in hours	Dose by injection equivalent to morphine injection 10 mg (single dose)	Dose by mouth equivalent to morphine injection 10 mg (single dose)
Morphine	2–4	10 mg	20–60 mg
Codeine	3	120 mg	200 mg
Fentanyl	4	100 mcg	N/A
Hydrocodone (Vicodin)	4	N/A	30–40 mg
Hydromorphone (Dilaudid)	3	2 mg	10 mg
Meperidine (Demerol)**	3	100 mg	300 mg
Methadone##	30	10 mg	10–20 mg
Oxycodone	3	N/A	20–30 mg
Propoxyphene (Darvocet)**	14	N/A	400 mg
Tramadol (Ultram)	6	Only the oral formulation of tramadol is available in the U.S. Low potency, not regulated as a "controlled drug" or "narcotic." Limited to 50–100 mg/dose and 400 mg/day due to seizure risk with higher doses.	

Elimination (t½) = the time required for elimination of 50% of the drug present.

** CNS toxicity of active metabolites limits use in chronic pain management.

Very long elimination time causes methadone to accumulate over many days. Because methadone is eliminated 10 times more slowly than morphine, with repeated dosing methadone is up to 10 time more potent than morphine and must be dosed with caution.

pain. Other than isolated case reports, there are no published data regarding the benefits or risks of using opioid analgesics for the control of chronic pain over the time course of several years.

There is no one "correct dose" of any given opioid that is safe and effective for all patients; the dosage must be titrated for each individual. The correct dose is one that reasonably controls pain with only minimal adverse effects. The required daily dose of an opioid can range over two to three orders of magnitude, depending on such factors as pain severity, the degree of opioid tolerance, and medical comorbidities.

With opioid analgesics, pain control must be balanced with minimal adverse effects

The use of opioid analgesics for control of acute pain is often limited by adverse effects of respiratory depression, sedation, nausea, pruritus (itching), urinary retention, and constipation. With the exception of constipation, patients tend to develop tolerance or resistance to these adverse effects with chronic use of opioid medications. Long-term use of opioids may be associated with additional adverse effects including:

- Impotence and loss of libido due to decreased release of sex hormones.
- Sweating and/or chills due to alteration of hormonal regulation of basal body temperature.
- Depression, although the overall risk of depression may be lessened if pain is controlled.
- Physical dependence.
- Opioid addiction.
- Tolerance (decreased effectiveness of a given dose of opioid to control pain).

Although the data are somewhat limited, mature adults with no history of drug or alcohol abuse appear to have only a low risk of developing addiction to opioid analgesics that are prescribed for the control of chronic pain. Prospective studies of pain patients suggest that the risk of a new onset of opioid addiction/dependence is between 1 in 100 and 1 in 1000. Given the high prevalence of substance abuse disorders in the general population, reactivation or worsening of existing substance abuse in patients treated with chronic opioid therapy is a much more common problem in clinical practice than are de novo cases of opioid addiction. Given the low risk of new addiction problems, concerns about addiction should not preclude consideration of opioid analgesics for the control of severe pain in mature adults who have no significant risk factors for substance abuse.

The risk of developing new addiction to opioid analgesics prescribed for pain is relatively low

It has long been clear that analgesic tolerance (i.e., decreased pain relief from a given dose) limits the utility of chronic opioid therapy. Although there is individual variability in the rate and extent to which tolerance develops, most patients who receive opioid analgesics for chronic pain over several weeks to many months, will require dosage escalation to achieve continued pain relief. The risk of developing opioid tolerance increases with the dose and duration of opioid therapy. Unfortunately, uncontrolled pain due to opioid tolerance may necessitate opioid dose escalation to regain pain control, and this in turn can cause further opioid tolerance. In order to keep the dosage as low as possible, in order to limit the development of tolerance and preserve the utility of opioid for future pain control, it may be necessary to employ a wide range of multidisciplinary pain therapies.

Chronic use of opioid analgesics for pain control may result in opioid tolerance hyperalgesia

One of the fundamental mechanisms of opioid tolerance appears to be that opioid analgesics not only inhibit, but paradoxically also facilitate or amplify, the neurotransmission of pain signals. With chronic administration of an opioid, the transmission of pain signals is enhanced, gradually and increasingly undermining the inhibitory (analgesic) effects of the medication. Although convincingly demonstrated in experimental animals, the significance of opioid tolerance-induced hyperalgesia in humans is unclear. However, methadone maintenance patients, and chronic pain patients requiring high doses of opioid, do have increased sensitivity to normally noxious stimuli (hyperalgesia). Minimizing, or even avoiding, the use of opioid analgesics appears to be the best way to avoid the development of opioid tolerance and opioid tolerance hyperalgesia.

Antidepressants and anticonvulsants are often used for treatment of neuropathic pain

Adjuvant analgesics, including several anticonvulsants, some antidepressants, and a few miscellaneous medications, have analgesic efficacy, especially in neuropathic pain. These adjuvant analgesics may be used alone or in combination with other opioid or nonopioid analgesics. In addition to pain relief, adjuvant analgesics may have other beneficial effects for chronic pain patients, including relief of insomnia, control of irritability, and, with antidepressants, management of comorbid depression and anxiety. The analgesic effects of many of the adjuvant analgesics have been extensively studied (Saarto & Wiffen, 2005; Wiffen, Collins, McQuay, Carroll, Jadad, & Moore, 2005). In general, these drugs have modest analgesic efficacy that, in some patients, may be offset by adverse effects. Despite such limitations, the adjuvant analgesics are important tools for chronic pain management.

Gabapentin, which is FDA approved for pain due to postherpetic neuralgia, is now widely used as a first-line analgesic for neuropathic pain. It is generally well tolerated and relatively free of drug-drug interactions that can complicate the use of other anticonvulsants. Common adverse effects, including sedation, cognitive impairment, and weight gain, are usually modest and resolve if the drug is discontinued. Treatment response is variable, with some individuals having marked pain improvement, and others receiving little or no benefit. The analgesic efficacy of gabapentin has been extensively studied for acute and chronic pain (Wiffen, McQuay, Edwards, & Moore, 2005).

Anticonvulsants must be tapered slowly due to a risk of new onset withdrawal seizures

Pregabalin (Lyrica) is a newer anticonvulsant that is thought to have similar mechanism of action as gabapentin. Although pregabalin appears to be a reasonably safe and effective adjuvant analgesic, to date there is no prospective data directly comparing the efficacy and safety of pregabalin with gabapentin. Other anticonvulsants, especially carbamazepine (Wiffen, McQuay, & Moore, 2005), have been used and extensively studied for pain control, but they must be used cautiously due to risks of adverse effects and drug-drug interactions. For example, some anticonvulsants including carbamazepine, oxcarbazepine, and topiramate increase hepatic metabolism of orally administered estrogens, potentially resulting in therapeutic failure of oral contraceptives. Anticonvulsants should be tapered over a period of one to two weeks, since abrupt discontinuation has been reported to be associated with new onset withdrawal seizures, even in patients with no prior seizure history.

Antidepressants are widely used in the management of chronic pain, due in part to the high prevalence of depression among patients with chronic pain. In addition to managing comorbid depression, some antidepressants have

Table 25
Adjuvant Analgesics for Use in Chronic Pain

Adjuvant analgesic	Generic name (trade name) Typical daily dose range	Considerations
Anticonvulsants		
	Gabapentin (Neurontin) 300–4800 mg/day	Sedation, dizziness are common AEs with anticonvulsants. Since abrupt discontinuation may precipitate withdrawal seizures, anticonvulsants should be tapered over 1–2 weeks.
		FDA approved for postherpetic neuralgia and widely used for neuropathic pain, increasingly used as a general analgesic, including for acute pain. AEs include weight gain. Few interactions with other drugs and no renal or hepatic toxicity. Cleared by the kidneys, so the dose must be markedly reduced in renal insufficiency.
	Pregabalin (Lyrica) 100–600 mg/day	FDA approved for postherpetic neuralgia and diabetic neuropathy pain. The mechanism is similar to gabapentin. AE includes weight gain. Few interactions with other drugs and no renal or hepatic toxicity. Cleared by kidneys, the dose must be markedly reduced in renal insufficiency.
	Carbamazepine (Tegretol) 100–1200 mg/day	Specifically used in trigeminal neuralgia, otherwise a second-line agent due to toxicity and drug interactions. Rare AEs include bone marrow suppression, skin rash/lesions, or hepatic toxicity which may be fatal. Decreases effectiveness of oral contraceptives.
	Lamotrigine (Lamictal) 50–400 mg/day	10% develop rash, but 1% develop severe (potentially fatal) skin reaction. Significant potential for drug interactions.
	Levetiracetam (Keppra) 500–3000 mg/day	AEs include fatigue, asthenia, depression. Few drug interactions.
	Oxcarbazepine (Trileptal) 300–2400 mg/day	Similar structure and mechanism as carbamazepine, but lower risk of most severe AEs. Decreases effectiveness of oral contraceptives.
	Tiagabine (Gabitril) 4–56 mg/day	Risk of onset of new seizure disorder. Other AEs include asthenia, confusion, abdominal pain.

Table 25 (continued)

Adjuvant analgesic	Generic name (trade name) Typical daily dose range	Considerations
	Topiramate (Topamax) 50–600 mg/day	AEs include weight loss (which some patients may view as beneficial), paresthesias, and kidney stones. Significant drug interactions. Decreases effectiveness of oral contraceptives.
	Zonisamide (Zonegran) 100–600 mg/day	AE include skin reactions (possibly fatal), photosensitivity, renal impairment, nephrolithiasis, abdominal pain, headache. Significant potential for drug interactions.
Antidepressants		May cause mania in susceptible individuals. Abrupt discontinuation may precipitate symptoms of depression, even when used for pain control.
Tricyclic antidepressants	Amitriptyline (Elavil) 10–300 mg/day	Generally more effective than SSRIs in neuropathic pain. AEs include constipation, dryness of mouth, weight gain, cardiac arrhythmias, urinary outlet obstruction, orthostatic hypotension (which may increase risk of falls in elderly). Use with methadone may increase risk of serious cardiac arrhythmia (QT prolongation). Extensively studied and widely used in management of neuropathic pain.
	Nortriptyline (Pamelor) 10–150 mg/day	A metabolite of amitriptyline associated with reduced risk of sedation, dryness of mouth, and/or weight gain.
	Imipramine (Tofranil) 10–300 mg/day	Similar utility to amitriptyline but with slightly less risk of sedation and/or dryness of mouth.
	Desipramine (Norpramin) 10–200 mg/day	A metabolite of imipramine associated with reduced risk of sedation, dryness of mouth, and/or weight gain.
Serotonin Norepinephrine Reuptake Inhibitors (SNRIs)	Duloxetine (Cymbalta) 30–120 mg/day	FDA approved for diabetic neuropathy. Two RCTs indicate analgesic effect in fibromyalgia. Avoid in renal failure, liver impairment, alcohol abuse. May worsen preexisting liver disease. Nausea, sedation, and dizziness are the most common AEs; significant weight loss is rare.

Table 25 (continued)

Adjuvant analgesic	Generic name (trade name) Typical daily dose range	Considerations
	Venlafaxine (Effexor) 75–375 mg/day	FDA approved for anxiety, and may be useful in headache, neuropathic pain, fibromyalgia. AEs include sedation, gastrointestinal upset, weight loss, tachycardia, hypertension, and QT prolongation. Frequency of sexual dysfunction similar to SSRIs.
Other antidepressants	Bupropion (Wellbutrin) 150–450 mg/day	One RCT suggests efficacy in neuropathic pain. Low risk of hypotension or sexual dysfunction. Seizure risk increases sharply with doses > 450 mg/day. Avoid if history of seizures. May be associated with weight loss.
Miscellaneous agents	Baclofen 15–80 mg/day	FDA approved for spasticity in multiple sclerosis and spinal cord lesions, also used for pain in these settings, and as a general muscle relaxant. A second-line agent for neuropathic pain, including trigeminal neuralgia. Sedation is a common AE. Seizures are more common if there is a history of stroke, brain injury, etc. Abrupt discontinuation may cause hallucinations, confusion, seizures.
	Tizanidine (Zanaflex) 4–36 mg/day	FDA approved for spasticity in multiple sclerosis and cerebral/spinal cord lesions, also used for pain in these settings, and as a general muscle relaxant. A second-line agent for neuropathic pain. Sedation and hypotension are the most common AEs. Fluvoxamine and ciprofloxacin markedly increase tizanidine levels and can produce severe hypotension. Hepatic enzyme elevation in 5% of patients; may lead to significant hepatotoxicity.

Abbreviations: AE = Adverse effects, FDA = U.S. Food and Drug Administration, OCD = Obsessive compulsive disorder, PTSD = posttraumatic stress disorder, t½ = elimination half-life (the time required for elimination of 50% of the drug present).

TCAs and SNRIs are more effective than SSRIs as analgesics

analgesic efficacy, at least in management of neuropathic pain (Saarto & Wiffen, 2005). The analgesic effect of tricyclics may be seen at doses lower than typically prescribed for treatment of depression. Amitriptyline is the best studied antidepressant in terms of pain relief, but other tricyclic antidepressants (nortriptyline, desipramine, etc.) also have analgesic efficacy. Cymbalta, a relatively new antidepressant, is FDA approved for control of pain due to diabetic peripheral neuropathy. There is less evidence supporting the use of SSRIs, but these agents are often reasonably well tolerated, and they should be considered if tricyclic antidepressants are poorly tolerated. The SSRIs may be especially useful in management of dysphoric mood and irritability that often accompanies chronic pain. Because the patient may be unaware of his or her increased irritability, it may be helpful to gain additional history from friends or family regarding the patient's mood and affect.

A treatment with perfect efficacy would have an NNT = 1

When comparing different medications or other therapies, a useful indicator of treatment efficacy is know as the "number needed to treat" (NNT). The NNT is an estimate of the total number of individuals that would have to be treated with a specific therapy for one individual to have the desired response, corrected for the placebo response rate. The formula for the NNT is:

$$NNT = \frac{1}{|P_a - P_c|}$$

where P_a is the probability of response to active therapy and P_c is the probability of response to placebo. Theoretically, treatments that are perfectly

Table 26
Estimated Number Needed to Treat (NNT) for Significant Improvement in Pain Intensity Score

Drug	Disease state	NNT (95% confidence interval)
Gabapentin*	PHN	3.9 (3.0–5.7)
Gabapentin*	DPN	2.9 (2.2–4.4)
Gabapentin*	Neuropathic pain	4.3 (3.5–5.7)
Carbamazepine**	TN	1.9 (1.4–2.8)
Carbamazepine**	Neuropathic pain	2.1 (1.5–2.7)
TCA***	DPN	1.3 (1.2–1.5)
TCA***	PHN	2.2 (1.7–3.1)
Amitriptyline***	Neuropathic pain	2.0 (1.7–3.1)

Number needed to harm (NNH) for minor adverse effect

Drug	Disease state	NNT (95% confidence interval)
Gabapentin*	Neuropathic pain	3.7 (2.4–5.4)
Carbamazepine**	Neuropathic pain	3.7 (2.4–7.8)
TCA***	Neuropathic pain	4.6 (3.3–36.7)

NNH for major adverse effect for carbamazepine was not significantly different that for placebo. This reflects that severe, but well known, adverse effects from carbamazepine are rare and simply did not occur in the study population.
Abbreviations: PHN = postherpetic neuralgia, DPN = diabetic peripheral neuropathy, TCA = tricyclic antidepressants.
* from Wiffen, McQuay, Edwards et al. (2005), ** from Wiffen, McQuay, & Moore (2005), *** from Saarto & Wiffen (2005).

efficacious would have NNT = 1, with every treated individual having the desired response. In practice, highly effective therapies may have a NNT of 2 or 3. Similarly, the risks of treatments may be compared by considering the number needed to harm (NNH). Treatments of relatively low efficacy (i.e., high NNT) may be reasonable choices when the potential benefit is significant and the NNH is also high (Cook & Sackett, 1995; McQuay & Moore, 1997). NNT and NNH can only be calculated from RCT data. Unfortunately, due to the difficulties in pain measurement, the wide range of clinical settings of chronic pain, and the diversity of available treatments, well-conducted RCTs are relatively uncommon in some areas of pain medicine. As a result, NNT and NNH values have been estimated only for a limited number of analgesics and treatment settings. It is only reasonable to compare NNT and NNH from different studies if the patient populations and the treatment responses measured in those studies are similar.

Interventional Therapies for Pain Management

Interventional therapies for chronic pain management include a wide range of surgeries, injections, and other procedures. Whereas analgesic medications often have broad indications in chronic pain, each interventional procedure is typically only indicated in specific situations. The goal of many interventional therapies, including most surgical procedures, is to correct, or at least modify, specific anatomic abnormalities, which were causing the pain. Other interventions, such as localized injections, are not designed to cure the underlying disease, but instead to decrease the neural transmission of pain signals. Local anesthetics and steroid injection therapies such as *trigger point injections* for muscular/myofascial pain or intraarticular joint injections for osteoarthritis may offer temporary relief (Bellamy, Campbell, Robinson, Gee, Bourne, & Wells, 2006). They are used to control severe exacerbations of chronic pain and to provide periods of pain relief designed to enable the patient to participate in physical therapy and rehabilitation. Excessive use of steroid-based injection therapies can lead to steroid toxicity, hyperglycemia, fluid retention, pituitary-adrenal suppression, osteoporosis, or Cushing's syndrome.

> Interventional therapies provide temporary pain relief to facilitate physical therapy

Since the indications for interventional therapies are specific to each technique, a pain specialist should be consulted if the patient does not respond to initial curative therapies, analgesics, or rehabilitation. Over the last 20 years, there has been a tremendous increase in the number of physicians specializing in the use of interventional procedures for the management of chronic pain. Such therapies are now available at most hospitals and in many office-based physician practices.

In general, *neurolytic techniques* to destroy nerve pathways transmitting pain signals are not appropriate for control of chronic, noncancer pain. Although permanent interruption of pain signal transmission might seem to be desirable in some cases, the risks of inadequate relief, worsened pain, and other iatrogenic effects of this approach are often prohibitive. Specific examples in which intentional neural destruction may be of benefit include radiofrequency ablation of spinal medial branch nerves and interventions for management of analgesic-resistant trigeminal neuralgia.

Spinal steroid injections (epidural steroid, selective nerve root or transforaminal epidural steroid) are a commonly used treatment for neck, back, and

Steroid injections reduce inflammation of spinal disks and facet joints

radiating arm or leg pain due to displaced intervertebral disks, spondylosis (degenerative arthritis of spine), spinal stenosis, or chronic pain after spine surgery. The long-term benefits of these procedures are modest, but they can provide short-term relief that can help to facilitate rehabilitation. The risk of needle trauma or spinal drug toxicity is very low, but similarly rare postinjection infections may have severe consequences including spinal cord damage and death. Spinal steroid injections and the other procedures listed below are minimally invasive and are usually performed on an outpatient basis.

Spinal facet joint injections and local anesthetic *medial branch nerve blocks* that innervate those joints, are indicated for pain due to facet arthropathy, i.e., osteoarthritis of the spinal facet joints. Facet arthropathy, or spinal spondylosis, is a common cause of axial neck and/or back pain, but there is little correlation between the severity of pain and the degree of joint abnormality seen on spinal radiographic imaging. Local anesthetic or steroid injections may help to corroborate the clinical diagnosis of facet arthropathy as the cause of pain, or to provide temporary pain relief to facilitate physical therapy. *Radiofrequency (RF) ablation* of the medial branch nerves is an important exception to the proscription against neural destruction to control noncancer pain. It can provide long periods (4–6 months) of relief of neck or back pain due to facet arthropathy (Niemisto, Kalso, Malmivaara, Seitsalo, & Hurri, 2003). If pain returns due to neural regeneration, the RF treatment can be repeated.

Neuromodulatory devices are considered only after less invasive treatments have been attempted

Implanted *spinal cord stimulators* and *peripheral nerve stimulators* are occasionally used for control of moderate to moderately-severe neuropathic pain that has not responded to analgesics. These implanted medical devices consist of an array of electrodes and an attached pulse generator (battery pack). The implanted stimulator can be controlled by an external programming device which communicates with the pulse generator via radiofrequency waves transmitted through the skin. With spinal cord stimulation, electrodes are positioned in the spinal canal, posterior to the spinal cord, so that electrical current through the device stimulates paresthesias in the areas affected by chronic pain. Peripheral

Neuropathic pain responds better to SCS than movement-related pain

nerve stimulators are similar implanted medical devices, with the stimulating electrodes implanted next to a peripheral nerve supplying the nerve input to the area of pain. Most patients perceive the stimulation paresthesias created by the stimulator as a tingling, warm, and soothing sensation that decreases pain intensity. The precise mechanism of pain relief is not known, but it probably involves spinal inhibition of pain signal transmission.

Peripheral nerve and spinal cord stimulation are usually modestly efficacious. Because neural stimulation may be ineffective if the patient has marked psychological or psychiatric comorbidity (Burchiel, Anderson, Wilson, Denison, Olson, & Shatin, 1995) candidates for implanted stimulation devices are usually referred for a preimplantation psychological evaluation. If no contraindications are identified during the psychological evaluation, the patient may subsequently undergo a temporary trial of stimulation therapy to determine its initial efficacy before permanent implantation of the stimulator device.

A spinal analgesic infusion pump is another pain control device for which patients may be referred for preimplant psychological assessment. Typically used for advanced cancer pain, spinal infusion pumps are also used for palliative care of otherwise intractable noncancer pain. Compared to systemic administration, spinal administration of a solution containing an opioid, local anesthetic, or other appropriate medication can provide more effective analgesia. The cost, complexity, and risks of spinal analgesics generally limit use to cases of truly intractable, incapacitating pain.

The decision whether to utilize an interventional therapy is based on a variety of disease and patient factors. For example, degenerative changes in the lower spine may result in narrowing of the spinal canal (i.e., lumbar spinal canal stenosis), which causes lower extremity pain from irritation of spinal nerves. Low intensity symptoms from mild stenosis may respond well to physical therapy or simple analgesics. Spinal injection therapies may help control exacerbations of pain or provide periods of pain relief and help facilitate physical therapy and rehabilitation. If the patient has severe spinal stenosis, spinal injections are more risky and less efficacious, so that surgical decompression of the spinal canal may be the best treatment option. If the patient declines surgical intervention, or is not a candidate for surgery due to increased risk of poor outcome due to comorbidities, additional trials of analgesics of other palliative pain therapies may be required. Optimal, individualized use of pain therapies may require the coordinated efforts of multiple healthcare professionals. Patients who do not respond to standard therapies are candidates for a multidisciplinary pain consultation, which is typically available through tertiary care medical centers.

4.3 Psychological Interventions

4.3.1 Cognitive-Behavioral Therapy

Psychological interventions for the treatment of chronic pain include a variety of approaches, the primary ones being: cognitive-behavioral therapy, behavioral or operant therapy, and self-regulatory therapies such as biofeedback,

> In this manual, CBT refers to a broad range of treatment approaches and techniques

---

Clinical Pearl
Elements of Cognitive-Behavioral Therapy

Behavioral elements:
- Changing the contingencies of reinforcement for pain behaviors (reinforcing well behaviors and extinguishing illness behaviors).
- Increasing "well behaviors" and behavioral activation through shaping and gradually increasing activity, goal setting, pacing and modifying activities, and skill training (e.g., communication skills, sleep hygiene, etc.).
- Reducing interpersonal and environmental contingencies and stimuli that reinforce pain behaviors.

Cognitive elements:
- Identifying and restructuring negative or unrealistic thoughts, expectations, beliefs, and attributions.
- Developing coping self-statements.

Self-regulatory elements:
- Relaxation, hypnosis, biofeedback, meditation, visual imagery.
- Attention diversion techniques.

relaxation, and hypnosis. With a cognitive-behavioral or behavioral approach, treatment may be provided within a limited definition of that therapeutic paradigm. For example, operant therapy may focus expressly on changing behaviors by changing contingencies of reinforcement, without incorporating elements of cognition therapy into the treatment. Similarly, cognitive-behavioral therapy may focus exclusively on beliefs, attributions, expectations, and dysfunctional cognitions without including behavioral or self-regulatory elements. However, in many programs, the term cognitive-behavioral therapy is a term that refers to a composite of cognitive-behavioral, operant, educational, and self-regulatory therapies. In the following sections on psychological intervention, the term cognitive-behavioral therapy (CBT) will refer to a broad range therapeutic approaches.

The specific components of cognitive-behavioral programs can vary with the nature of the program and/or the needs of the individual patient. There are however, core components that are usually included in most CBT programs for chronic pain.

- *Education:* An introduction to pain transmission and modulation that includes examples of biological, psychological and social factors that influence pain perception.
- *Goal-setting:* Individual long-term and short-term goals.
- *Relaxation techniques:* As strategies for self-management of pain, to manage stress, reduce muscle tension, aid in distraction from pain, and help with sleep.
- *Skill acquisition:* To improve communication skills, learn activity pacing, develop stress management strategies, and good sleep hygiene.
- *Cognitive:* Identify and modify pain-related cognitions, attributions, beliefs, fears, and expectations, and develop pain-coping statements.
- *Maintenance:* Identify or strengthen the patient's social support network, anticipate problems, and develop strategies for coping with setbacks and relapses.
- *Exercise:* General conditioning and proper body mechanics to address deconditioning, poor endurance, and fatigue. This part of the program is usually led by a physical therapist.

CBT may be inpatient or outpatient, individual or group

CBT may be provided alone or with other treatments such as physical therapy and/or medical therapies. It may be offered as an inpatient or outpatient service, and in individual or group formats. Advantages of individual CBT include the opportunity for a therapist to give his or her undivided attention to the patient and to tailor the treatment to the patient's specific needs. Group sessions have the advantages of social interaction, peer support, sharing of ideas, modeling of adaptive behaviors, and opportunities for mutual validation of experiences.

The patient's treatment goals and expectations should be discussed at the first session. The therapist should work collaboratively with the patient to develop a set of mutually acceptable goals. This can help to prevent feelings of frustration, anger, and failure if the patient's initial expectations, such as complete relief from pain, are not met. Treatment goals may vary across psychological treatment approaches (e.g., operant, cognitive, cognitive-behavioral, family), as well as across the various disciplines that may be involved in the patient's care. Providers, patients, referral sources, and family members may have different treatment goals. Whereas a successful outcome for a particular patient might be significant pain reduction, the health care providers may be looking for functional gains and decreased medication use. An employer may want the patient to return to work, and the family may be hoping for a return to a sense of normalcy.

Unrealistic patient goals can sabotage treatment

Having patients complete homework assignments between sessions helps integrate therapeutic material into everyday life. Pain diaries also work well as homework. They can help patients recognize fluctuations in pain and track variables that influence those fluctuations such as changes in weather, over- or underactivity, strong emotions, stress, etc. Patients can use diaries to record their responses to increases in pain. Responses might include taking medication, resting, using heat or ice, stretching, distraction, or using relaxation or meditation techniques. Pain diaries can reveal whether the patient is relying on just one or two coping strategies or is developing a broader range of pain coping techniques. An example of a pain diary is included in the Appendix.

Homework helps patients incorporate coping skills into everyday lives

4.3.2   Education

Education about theories of pain is an interesting, and in many ways necessary, starting point for therapy. Patients are often quite interested in learning about how theories of pain transmission, and the understanding of pain perception and expression, have evolved over the centuries. Additionally, discussing this

---

Clinical Vignette
Modulation of Pain Perception

Attention and pain modulation
- "If you have a toothache, when does it hurt most? Often at night when you try to sleep because there is nothing to take your attention away from the pain."
- "If you're watching a good movie or are engrossed in conversation with a friend, you may be less aware of your pain. Pain shifts from foreground to background depending on where your attention is focused."

Attention directed toward pain increases pain perception

Cognition and pain modulation
- "If you believe that the pain in your chest signifies problems with your heart, you're likely to feel fear or anxiety and call your doctor. If you think the pain in your chest means that you ate too much for dinner, you may merely be irritated with yourself and take an antacid."
- "If you believe that pain controls you, you're likely to feel angry and frustrated and give up trying. If you believe that you have some degree of control over pain, you are likely to feel more hopeful and optimistic."

Cognitions influence affective and behavioral responses to pain

Affect and pain modulation
- "When you're feeling down, depressed, irritable, or angry, pain seems worse than at times when your mood is upbeat and positive."
- "If you "get up on the wrong side of the bed" and start the day off with an argument with your spouse, your pain will probably be more intense than on a day when you feel loved and cared for by your friends and family."

Education about pain transmission allows for discussion of the multiple factors that inhibit and facilitate pain

topic enables the therapist to present Melzack and Wall's (1965) gate-control theory and to introduce the concept of the multiple dimensions of pain. (A summary of theories may be found in Chapter 2. Additional sources of information about theories of pain are listed in the resources section.) Learning about gate control theory helps the patient to understand pain signal detection and transmission, facilitation and inhibition of signal transmission, pain perception, and the difference between injury and pain. When discussing the "gate," and how various factors can modulate pain, it can be helpful to start with an example of how pain transmission may be inhibited:

Introduce the concept of pain signal inhibition with an everyday example

> When you bang your elbow in the doorway and feel a shooting pain, the usual response is to rub your elbow. When you do this, your pain decreases. This is because the nerve fibers that send "touch" information to the brain inhibit or dampen down pain signal transmission. The injury doesn't change, but the "gate" closes.

When introducing how psychological factors modulate pain, discuss the multiple dimensions of pain (sensory, cognitive, and emotional) as proposed by Melzack and Casey (1968). These dimensions are interrelated; changes in one dimension influence the others. Changes in affective states, attention, beliefs, and cognitions can influence both pain perception and pain coping.

4.3.3   Identifying and Restructuring Negative Cognitions

CBT treats the negative thoughts, beliefs, and attributions that accompany pain

Cognitive theory and therapy, as developed by Aaron Beck in 1976, was initially a means of understanding and treating depression. Identifying, challenging, and restructuring dysfunctional thoughts and core beliefs (or schemas) are some of the most important tools of cognitive therapy. In the pain management setting, identifying and challenging dysfunctional pain-related thoughts, attributions, expectations and beliefs about pain is the focus of therapy. An excellent resource for a cognitive approach to the management of chronic pain is Beverly Thorn's *Cognitive Therapy for Chronic Pain*: *A Step-by-Step Guide* (2004).

Clinical Pearl
Identifying and Restructuring Negative Cognitions

1. Start with an everyday example.
"You're on your way to the store, stop at a stop sign, and begin to pull into the intersection. The driver on your left runs the stop sign and you slam on the brakes to avoid an accident. You might say "Boy, that jerk makes me mad! We could have been hurt or killed." The other driver's actions cause you to be angry – right? There is something else that happens between the event (braking) and the emotion (anger). Any idea what that is?"
Explain the relationship between thoughts and emotions with examples of how different cognitions result in different emotional responses.

2. Present a pain-related example.
"You have a lunch date planned with a friend at noon but when you get up in the morning, your pain is worse than usual."

Clinical Pearl (continued)

When discussing the relationship between thoughts and emotions, you might ask the patient's emotional response to this scenario and work backward to the intervening thought. Or you might begin with thoughts and discuss how the emotional response varies depending on the cognition.

3. Discuss cognitive distortions such as catastrophizing, all or nothing thinking, "should" statements and discounting the positives and how they influence coping with pain.
> **"Should" statement:** "I should be able to clean the house in one day like I did before."
> **Emotion:** Frustration, anger.
> **Restructured statement:** "I can't do things like I did before, but if I do a little bit everyday, I can still manage to keep the house looking neat."
> **Emotion:** Hopefulness.

4. Have patients provide examples from their own experience, identify and work through them, restructuring negative and/or dysfunctional cognitions.

5. Give homework assignments for identifying negative thoughts and emotional and behavioral responses to these thoughts. Ask the patient to develop alternative, more adaptive ways of thinking about situations or events. Take time to review homework to assure that patients incorporate ideas, to correct misunderstandings and assess progress

6. Coping self-statements are those statements that help the patient cope more adaptively with pain and stressful situations. They are not statements of wishful thinking or denial of reality. They acknowledge the difficulty of the situation yet reflect a realistic and balanced perspective. For example, when faced with an exacerbation of pain, an example of a coping self-statement might be,
> "I've been through this before and it will pass. If I take a hot shower, do a little stretching, and use meditation it will probably be better by this afternoon."
> Positive coping statements can be developed and used to replace negative thoughts as they are identified.

Positive self-statements are used to replace negative and dysfunctional thoughts

4.3.4 Changing Behaviors

In the early 1970s, Wilbur Fordyce developed a behaviorally oriented pain management program at the University of Washington in Seattle based on B.F. Skinner's model of behavioral conditioning. Using the concepts of *operant conditioning,* Fordyce's program focused on changing pain behaviors by modifying environmental contingencies. The principals of operant conditioning suggest that positively (or negatively) reinforced behaviors will increase, while behaviors that are punished or not reinforced (extinguished) will decrease. Fordyce proposed that pain behaviors are subject to operant conditioning, and that behaviors which communicate the presence of pain increase or decrease in response not only to variations in the severity of pain, but also in response to reinforcement contingencies.

Wilbur Fordyce proposed that pain behaviors could be modified by changing reinforcement contingencies

Negative reinforcement eliminates a negative event or effect

Pain behaviors include:
- Verbal communications (complaints, moaning, groaning).
- Motor behaviors (limping, guarding).
- Activity level (time spent sitting or lying down).
- Requests for assistance or pain medications.

Fordyce suggested that these behaviors could be positively reinforced (thereby increasing their chance of occurring) by the responses of family, friends, and health care providers, financial incentives, and the administration of pain medications. For example, verbal complaints may result in increased attention from a spouse, or in the administration of as-needed pain medications. If spousal attention, or the provision of pain medication, are contingent on the patient's overt pain behaviors (i.e., they are more likely to occur when the patient engages in the behavior than when he or she does not), they can reinforce this behavior (i.e., increase its frequency).

In the behavioral treatment paradigm, contingencies are modified such that "well" behaviors as opposed to "illness" (or pain) behaviors are reinforced. "Uptime," that is time spent engaging in activity such as household chores, socializing or exercising, is positively reinforced. Pain behaviors are subjected to extinction, that is, the removal of positive or negative reinforcement maintaining each specific pain behavior. In behavioral programs, pain medication is provided on a time-contingent, versus an "as needed," schedule to reduce the positive reinforcing quality of pain medications. Exercise is performed to "success" rather than to "tolerance" as an end-point, that is, patients stop exercising when a specified number of repetitions (or period of time) have been achieved, as opposed to stopping when pain increases. In this way rest serves as positive reinforcement, successful completion of exercise, rather than as a negative reinforcement, avoidance of pain. Treatment of chronic pain in the operant conditioning paradigm includes gradually increasing well behaviors through positive reinforcement, shaping and gradual change; the use of extinction to reduce pain behaviors; and reducing interpersonal and environmental stimuli that maintain pain behaviors.

Goal Setting

Setting and completing goals allows patients to gradually engage in a desired behavior or activity through reasonable and attainable steps. Long-term goals incorporate short-term goals which the patient believes can be accomplished within an agreed upon time frame. Short-term goals may be modified in therapy sessions if the patient finds them too challenging or too easily achievable. During the first session, help patients develop long-term and short-term goals. Long-term goals might include areas such as exercise, educational or vocational progress, household tasks, socialization, and recreational activities. Goals should be:

1. *Realistic.* For a patient who has had three back surgeries and continues to experience pain, the goal of running a marathon is not realistic. A realistic goal for such a patient might be to start or to increase the frequency of appropriate conditioning exercise.
2. *Desirable.* Most pain patients have long lists of chores and tasks they "should" be accomplishing. However, therapeutic success – especially early in the course of CBT – often depends upon choosing desirable goals rather than ones that the patient considers to be "necessary."
3. *"Patient-centered."* Therapeutic goals should be achievable by the patient and should depend as little as possible on other people's actions.

Short-term goals are the intermittent steps the patient will have to take in order to achieve the long-term goals. If, for example, the patient's long-term goal is to be less socially isolated, calling a friend to go to lunch or a movie would be a realistic initial short-term goal. Developing and reviewing goals presents therapy as an active, collaborative process between therapist and patient.

When therapy is conducted in a group setting, the congratulations of other group members often serve as positive reinforcement for goal-directed behaviors. However, it is also important that patients learn to provide themselves with positive reinforcement for steps completed toward long-term goals. Patients often have difficulty acknowledging small steps as successes. They compare their present abilities with what they were capable of accomplishing in the past and often judge themselves as coming up short. It may be necessary to discuss why present accomplishments are as important as those achieved in the past. Family members can be recruited to acknowledge and congratulate the successful completion of goals.

Patients need to positively reward themselves for successful completion of goals

Pacing Daily Activities

Patients exhibit a broad range of responses to chronic pain and to the physical limitations it often imposes. At one extreme are patients who spend much of the day in bed or on the couch, fearful of moving, and dwelling on their pain. At the other end of the spectrum are patients who "refuse to give in" to their pain and attempt to maintain their normal schedule as though they did not have pain. More often, one finds patients who restrict everyday activity and then have bursts of activity on "good" days. These are the patients who will clean the house, mow the lawn, or weed the garden on days when their pain is less severe than usual. Such bursts of activity are often followed by several days spent "down" or in bed. Developing activity-pacing skills helps patients to maintain a sustainable schedule of activity instead of bouncing back and forth between too much and too little.

Patient activity is often like a "yo-yo" – up one day and down the next

Pacing can either be a matter of increasing or limiting daily activity. If a patient engages in very limited daily activity, the goal will be to develop a slowly but steadily increasing schedule of activity. If the patient engages in a "yo-yo" pattern of activity, bouncing between too much and too little, the goal will be to develop a more consistent schedule. In their excellent, patient-focused manual, *Manage Your Pain,* Michael Nicholas and his colleagues (2000) developed the following suggestions for pacing.

Pacing entails understanding one's limitations in order to make adjustments in activities

1. On a scale of 0 to 10 (with 0 being *no pain* and 10 being *worst imaginable pain*) allow pain to increase no more than 2 points while engaging in any task. If the task increases pain more than 2 points, decrease the amount of time spent on it, or modify the task so that it is less challenging.
2. Regulate the amount of time spent doing each activity in order to keep pain within the 2-point range. For example, if loading the dishwasher increases pain beyond 2 points, try loading only half of the dishwasher. If loading half of the dishwasher maintains pain within the 2-point range, then half of the dishwasher becomes the base for that activity. Vacuuming is another example. If, after several attempts, vacuuming one room maintains pain within the 2-point limit, then vacuuming one room becomes the base for that activity.
3. Write each task on a Post-it® note and indicate how much can be completed while staying within the 2-point limit. For example, vacuuming: one room;

ironing: 2 pieces; mowing the yard: ½ of the yard; folding one category of laundry (towels, for example).

4. Plan each day with a combination of necessary tasks (active and sedentary), periods of rest, stretching and exercises, and some pleasurable activities, e.g., meeting a friend for lunch or a movie.

5. Arrange the Post-it® notes to plan a day's activities. For example:

   1. Loading half of the dishwasher (standing and bending) followed by...
   2. Opening the mail and paying bills (seated, limited physical demands) followed by...
   3. 10 minutes of stretching, followed by...
   4. Errands (driving and walking), followed by...
   5. 20–30 minutes of meditation or relaxation, etc.

Activity pacing lends itself well to homework assignments and review

Communication Skills

People understand acute pain, few have an understanding of chronic pain

Learning good communication skills can be very helpful for patients with chronic pain. Because others in their daily lives often do not, and really cannot, understand their experience of chronic pain, patients can end up feeling isolated, misunderstood, and resentful. Although patients may be constantly aware of their pain, it is not always apparent to others. It falls to the patients themselves to communicate how they are feeling and why they are feeling that way, why their ability to be active fluctuates, and what their needs are (assistance, emotional support, time alone, distraction, etc.).

As patients become more active, get involved with exercise, care for their appearance, lose weight, etc., others may perceive them as no longer "ill" or limited. Friends, family, and acquaintances may believe that the patient has "recovered" and have little understanding about continuing pain or the effort required to remain active and effectively manage it. The patient may hear comments such as, "Well, if you can (mow the yard, volunteer at church, take a walk, etc.) then why can't you work?" or "I don't understand why you can't (take in a movie, go shopping, etc.) today. You did it last week." or "But you look fine." These can be difficult situations for patients to respond to in ways that are not angry or defensive. Patients often report feeling that others perceive them as "faking" or "lazy," and such remarks can lead to resentment, distancing, and feelings of isolation. This can be a very fruitful area to explore, as patients are often able to come up with many examples from their own experience.

Patients can learn to communicate what they need from others without anger, blame, or resentment

When patients say, "They (i.e., my family, friends, coworkers, etc.) don't understand!" an appropriate response is, "You're right, they don't." Everyone has had experience with acute pain, and this is how most people understand pain. Pain is supposed to resolve when the injury has healed. Few people have experience with, or an understanding of, chronic pain. Sessions that focus on effective communication help patients learn how to help others understand chronic pain and how to communicate their needs. Too often, patients inadvertently raise barriers to communication by making statements such as, "I just wish you could have my pain for five minutes – then maybe you'd understand it!" or "I just can't...because I'm in pain." Sessions spent on developing effective pain-related communications strive to help patients achieve the following aims:

- Understand that others cannot read his or her mind (or body).
- Understand that educating family and friends about chronic pain and physical limitations becomes the responsibility of the patient.
- Understand and communicate needs when pain is severe or when assistance is required.
- Develop ways to turn conversation away from pain, as continual focus on pain can alienate others.
- Develop a communication style that is direct, that addresses the problem at hand, and that is not excessively confrontive or blaming.

Clinical Vignette
Communication Skills

Communicating intent:
Your family doesn't have the awareness of your pain that you have – they can't "see" it. If you're with your family watching TV in the evening and suddenly get up and leave the room to go lie down, they don't know why you left. They may attribute all kinds of (incorrect) motives to your leaving, e.g., they may think you're angry or upset. One simple sentence such as, "I'm really hurting right now and need to go lie down," clearly communicates your intention.

Communicating needs:
Family and friends often have difficulty seeing a loved one in pain. They may want to help but don't know how. If they know that you're hurting, but don't know how to be helpful, they may end up feeling resentful that they can't "fix" the problem for you. Rather than just saying that you're hurting, let others know what you need – it may be a backrub, someone to watch a movie with you to distract you from pain, time alone, or just someone to listen. One patient told her husband "You don't need to fix it, I just need you to listen for a minute."
If others are overly solicitous, providing assistance you don't really need, you can end up feeling more disabled than you are. Others can be so helpful that you end up with little meaningful activity during your day. Consider addressing your family or friends with something like the following: "I know you're really trying to help me with all you do. But I end up feeling useless sometimes, and I'd like to do what I can for myself, whenever possible. When I need your help, I'll ask. It's good to know I can call on you."

Knowing when and how to direct conversation away from pain:
Others may believe that it's the polite thing to do to always begin a conversation (or the day) with asking how you feel. Over time, you become known as your pain problem. As one patient said, "That's me. I'm 'The Back'." It falls to you to let others know that you're not limited to discussing pain, that you have other interests and would like to talk about them. For example, if a friend always ask how your (pain problem) is, you may say something like "Thanks for asking but my (pain problem) always hurts... I have chronic pain. Let's talk about (topic of your choice) instead."

> Patients need to know when and how to redirect conversation away from pain

An excellent resource for developing effective communication can be found in Barbara Pachter's book *The Power of Positive Confrontation* (2000). In it, she describes a series of steps for effective communication in difficult situations:

- *What* is bothering you? Define the problem in a specific, simple way that avoids negatively labeling the other person.

Clinical Vignette
Addressing Difficult Confrontations

Problem: A friend asks how you are, and you remark that you're having a bad pain day. She says (rather incredulously), "You *still* have that pain?"

What: "When you say it like that I feel defensive – like I have to justify having pain. Chronic pain is part of my life – sometimes its better and sometimes its worse."

Ask: "As my friend I hope you will try to understand and not dismiss that part of my life."

Check in: "Can I count on you?"

Problem: You are making the bed and wince as you pull up the cover. Your husband sees this and says, "Honey, you go sit down. You don't need to be doing that – I'll finish."

What: "I think I can make the bed and need to remain as active as possible. I need to feel like a contributing person in the family."

Ask: "I'd like to do as much as I can but hope that I can count on your help if I ask."

Check in: "Is that OK with you?"

- *Ask* for what is it you would like the person you're addressing to do. Make certain your request is possible for the other person and state it in a simple, direct manner.
- *Check in* by asking a simple question to assure you've been understood and if your request can happen, e.g., "OK?" or "Can you do that?"

Using this formula, it is possible to address a variety of difficult situations with friends, family, acquaintances, and coworkers. Clear, positive, and accurate communication may not always produce the desired results, but it at least allows requests to be stated without anger or blame, and increases the likelihood of being heard and understood.

Sleep Hygiene

Insomnia can be influenced by medication, depression, anxiety, and poor sleep habits

Poor sleep commonly co-occurs with chronic pain. Pain can contribute to disrupted and nonrestorative sleep. For example, patients often report that pain wakes them up when they are changing position. Poor sleep may also be attributable to depression, or to medications. Some medications, particularly opioids, have been found to decrease the deep stages of sleep. The combination of poor sleep, unstructured days, and opioids often results in patients sleeping or nodding off during the day. In some cases, the patient's normal circadian cycles of behavior may be inverted. Being up at night and sleeping during the day results in even fewer opportunities to interact with others and to engage in normal daytime activities.

Good sleep hygiene can help improve sleep

Clinical Pearl:
Treatment Considerations for Sleep Problems

1. **Medications.** Are pain medications contributing to poor sleep and, if so, can they be adjusted? Should an antidepressant, such as low dose amitriptyline or trazodone, be considered to help with sleep? These medications can be prescribed by a psychiatrist, primary care physician, or pain specialist.

Clinical Pearl (continued)

2. **Sleep habits.** Has the patient developed poor sleep habits, such as taking extended naps during the day or watching TV until falling asleep late at night? Developing good sleep hygiene can help improve sleep.

3. **Depression.** Is depression contributing to poor sleep? Depression occurs in approximately half of all patients seen for chronic pain, so it should always be evaluated and treated when present. Antidepressants should be considered, particularly as some are also analgesics (amitriptyline, duloxetine) and others assist with sleep (amitriptyline, trazodone). Issues that contribute to depression such as losses, functional limitations, feelings of guilt or worthlessness, or fears about the future, should be addressed in therapy sessions.

4. **Stress and worry.** Are worries about finances, employment, or marital problems interfering with good sleep? As with depression, stressors and worries contributing to poor sleep should be addressed in therapy. These problems may be amenable to cognitive therapy, marital therapy, or stress management. For patients who have insomnia due to worrying, consider the following suggestions:
   (a) Write down plans for the next day (or week) and current worries at a speci-fied time, for no longer than 30 minutes.
   (b) Stop worrying, planning, etc. for 30 minutes before bedtime.
   (c) Keep a pad and pencil next to the bed to jot down a reminder if awakened by worries during the night.

Clinical Pearl
Hints to the Patient for Developing Good Sleep Habits

Keep a regular schedule.
- A regular sleep schedule entails going to bed at the same time and getting up at the same time even if sleep was poor the previous night.
- Use an alarm. The goal is to regulate sleep over the long run.

Avoid lengthy daytime naps.
- Rest or practice relaxation several times each day, but avoid extended naps (longer than 30 minutes), which can interfere with nighttime sleep.

Use the bedroom for sleep and sex only.
- No TV, crossword puzzles, eating, or talking on the phone while in bed. This helps develop a mental connection between the place and the purpose.
- Avoid late night meals, caffeinated beverages, heavy snacks with high fat or sugar content, and heavy alcohol intake. A glass of wine, herbal tea, or a carbohydrate rich snack such as half a bagel, may help with falling sleep.

Relax 30 minutes before retiring.
- Consider a relaxing activity before going to bed such as:
  - Taking a warm bath.
  - Drinking an herbal tea, milk, or warm milk.
  - Reading a magazine or book (avoid 'page-turners').
  - Watching a TV program.
  - Listening to soothing music.

4.3.5   Self-Regulatory Techniques

Patients can benefit from learning how to use self-management techniques for managing chronic pain. These include: diaphragmatic breathing, progressive and passive relaxation, imagery, autogenic phrases, hypnosis, meditation, and biofeedback. Although each technique has distinctive elements, all of them aim to reduce stress, increase physical relaxation, and focus attention.

Relaxation is a skill that requires practice and patience to learn

When relaxation is introduced as a technique for managing pain, some patients mistakenly assume that they are essentially being told that their pain is "in your head," or that it is "caused" by stress, anxiety, or depression. It is important to assure patients that you believe that their pain is real. It is also important to clarify what relaxation-based techniques can and cannot do. They are not panaceas. They will not cure, or eliminate pain. They can help to decrease chronic pain, even if only briefly, and they can help the patient cope with the stress of living with chronic pain.

Breathing Techniques

Slow, deep breathing can help refocus attention, slow metabolism, and reduce tension

Slow, deep breathing is one of the most basic relaxation techniques, and it is often the starting point for teaching more advanced relaxation techniques. Simple breath relaxation involves nothing more complex than a passive focus on breathing – noticing the inhale/exhale cycle, or the rise and fall of the chest or belly. A more active breathing technique is diaphragmatic breathing or "belly breathing" which entails pulling air deep into the torso. Many people overuse the upper body when breathing and find it difficult to redirect their breath. In order to locate the muscles that will expand when breathing diaphragmatically, have the patient place the palm of his or her hand on the "round" part of the belly and, with a sharp rapid intake of breath, make the hand "jump." This movement helps locate the muscles recruited with diaphragmatic breathing. Leaving a hand on the round part of the belly helps a patient feel the expansion and contraction that occurs when the diaphragm is being actively engaged. Some patients are able to learn diaphragmatic breathing techniques in a single session; others may need several sessions of guided

---

Clinical Pearl
Hints to the Patient for Practicing Relaxation

- Find a quiet room without noise or distractions. Turn off the phone and the TV, and set aside 20–30 minutes for uninterrupted time alone.

- Sit in a comfortable chair that supports the head and arms. Try not to lie prone, especially on a bed, as it is easy to fall asleep when relaxed.

- Loosen tight clothing such as belts, shoes, and ties, and remove glasses.

- The art of relaxation requires attention, practice, and consistency. Set aside time each day to practice relaxation, whether it is for 15, 20, or 40 minutes. Some days, a relaxation exercise goes well, and feels wonderful and refreshing; other days, it can be more difficult to relax and keep attention focused on breathing. Whether or not the relaxation practice session goes well, stay with it. A difficult session doesn't mean that it won't become easier and more effective with time and practice.

Clinical Pearl
Hints to the Therapist for Guiding a Relaxation Exercise

- Pace your speech. Speak slowly, rhythmically, and distinctly. Pause from time to time. Speak with a "hypnotic" tone of voice, which is somewhat lower in pitch, has less conversational inflection, and is soothing and reassuring.

- Use short sentences and informal speech.

- Use repetition. Phrases such as "breathe in deeply...breathe out slowly" or "Let your (arms, legs, hands, etc.) feel heavy, comfortable, and relaxed" can be repeated many times during the exercise.

practice. An excellent description of breathing techniques for relaxation can be found in Jon Kabat-Zinn's *Full Catastrophe Living* (1990).

While the patient focuses on his or her breathing, several things occur that aid relaxation. Attention narrows, whether the focus is passive observation or learning a specific breathing technique. With a narrowed attentional field, pain may begin to shift from foreground to background. As respiration slows and the state of relaxation deepens, muscle tension lessens. With further slowing of respiration, the metabolism slows.

Following is an example of a relaxation exercise beginning with a passive focus on breathing, progressing to diaphragmatic breathing.

Clinical Pearl
Example of Relaxation Exercise

Place your feet flat on the floor. Let your arms fall comfortably in your lap or be supported on the arms of the chair. Let your body feel comfortable and well supported by the chair. Close your eyes. Now, let your attention go to your breath... let go of all other thoughts and distractions and just notice what it feels like to breathe in...and breathe out. Just breathe naturally...notice the rise and fall of your chest, your belly as you breathe in...and breathe out. Let your breathing drop into a slow, natural rhythm. Watching your breath can be like watching the waves at the beach...they flow in...and they flow out. Watching your breath is much like watching waves...one is slow and full...another is less deep...whatever happens is just fine. Now, place your hand flat on your belly...it doesn't matter which hand. As you breathe in, bring your air all the way down into your belly...let it fill like a balloon. Feel the expansion of the air in your belly...feel your belly swell up...and out. Notice how your ribs expand as you inhale...and contract as you exhale. When you exhale...exhale slowly...take your time and let your air all the way out. You may want to purse your lips lightly so you can feel your air slowly release. Breathe out slowly...all the way down...all the way out.

When you get to the bottom of your breath, there's a moment when you're not breathing in...and you're not breathing out...it's just quiet. When you get here, just wait. Don't hold your breath, but pause...just wait for your next breath....wait for your body to breathe you. Breathe in deeply...breathe out slowly.

Progressive and Passive Relaxation

Progressive and passive relaxation are widely used relaxation techniques. *Progressive relaxation* entails alternately tensing and relaxing muscles. For example, the muscles in the right hand and forearm arm are tensed and held in a tensed position for a specified period of time, often four counts. The tension is then released and the muscles allowed to relax. During this time the difference between the tensed state and the relaxed state is observed. Tensing and releasing is repeated through different muscle groups. Although this is an excellent technique for learning relaxation, chronic pain patients often have significant muscle tension stemming from the original injury, or secondarily from guarding. If the tensing phase of progressive relaxation exacerbates pain, consider using a passive technique.

Passive relaxation involves observing a particular muscle, or group of muscles, and allowing it to relax and release tension. Whereas with progressive relaxation a person can fairly readily learn to distinguish tense from relaxed states, it can be more difficult to learn to release tension from a resting muscle. Observing the natural release of tension and muscle relaxation that occurs while exhaling can be a helpful technique when learning to relax. Once the patient has learned to breath slowly and deeply, whether with diaphragmatic breathing or by allowing his or her breath to slow naturally over time, passive observation of various muscle groups during the exhale can help with learning the sensations associated with relaxation.

> **Clinical Pearl**
> **Example of Passive Relaxation**
>
> Let your attention go to your feet and ankles...just notice how they feel...the heaviness...the weight of your feet against the floor. Now let your breath out slowly...slowly and completely...and as you breath out notice the feelings in your feet and ankles. You may be aware of heaviness...not just heaviness but a profound sense of weight, as if your feet were bricks or heavy pieces of metal.
>
> You could move them if you wanted...but they feel too comfortable and too heavy to bother. You may notice feelings of tingling...or warmth...or you may notice other sensations. It doesn't matter what it is you feel and observe...just be aware of feelings in your feet and ankles as you breathe out slowly and completely. (Move observation to other muscles – often moving up through the body. For example from the feet and ankles, to the calves, then thighs, hips, lower back, and so on.)

Meditation

Meditation is related to relaxation in that breathing will be slow and regular and muscles relaxed. It adds to physical relaxation the dimension of mental quieting and stillness, and a focus on the present moment. Learning how to relax the body is comparatively straightforward, and the concept of physical relaxation is familiar to most patients. Keeping the mind still is less straightforward, and learning this skill is not integral to Western culture. In societies in which productivity and activity are highly valued, stillness and inactivity are discouraged. Some patients will not agree to use meditation techniques unless the clinician first works with them to overcome this cultural barrier. Some patients are unwilling to engage in relaxation techniques because of their religious beliefs. It may help to discuss how prayer, which requires mental stillness and focus, is similar to meditation. Patients may be willing to use prayer

Clinical Pearl
Hints to the Therapist for Teaching Meditation

- Have the patient begin meditation wearing comfortable clothes and sitting in a **comfortable position,** without any distractions.

- Suggest that the amount of time to be spent meditating be decided before beginning. A meditation may begin with short periods of time, ten or fifteen minutes, and gradually increase to 30 to 45 minute meditations.

- Begin meditation by having the patient develop **slow, regular breathing** either using diaphragmatic breathing or merely allowing the breath to slow over time.

- Following is an example of how the passive, nonjudgmental focus of meditation can be guided.

  Find a **focus point.** You may focus on the breath... being aware of breathing in...and breathing out. Or consider using a simple, neutral word like the word "One." You may use a word like "Peace"... or "Re—lax." This serves as a mental anchor, which can help keep the mind on the moment rather than drifting off to sea. As thoughts come to mind...and they will..., sounds come into awareness...or physical sensations become apparent, notice them... but let them go. Return your attention to your focus point. This is the **passive, nonjudgmental attitude** of meditation. Thoughts cross the mind... sounds and sensations compete for your attention,...but nothing requires a response from you. Thoughts come...and they go. It's like watching them on a screen...or watching someone else's thoughts or feelings. They require no response from you...just let them go.

- Although meditation entails a state of passive and nonjudgmental focus on the immediate moment, it is not easy to learn. Like all skills, it requires practice, and it will go well sometimes and not so well at other times.

- Remind the patient not to critically judge his or her performance or to assume that it's not working if the mind wanders. This is the natural process of learning the practice of meditation.

as their form of meditation. However, if a patient is clearly uncomfortable with relaxation and meditation consider using a different method to learn relaxation, such as biofeedback.

Meditation is related to breathing slowly and regularly; the breath itself may serve as the focal point for attention. Meditation adds a nonjudgmental attitude toward thoughts and perceptions that try to draw attention away from the focus on the moment. The aim of meditation is to remain focused only on the moment at hand, without thinking about the past or planning or worrying about the future.

There are many forms of meditation. Other examples can be found in books by Jon Kabat-Zinn (1990) and Shinzen Young (2004).

Autogenic Training

Autogenic training was developed by J.H. Schultz and Wolfgang Luthe (1959). Their techniques were developed from observations of patients during hypnosis. While hypnotized, patients reported physical sensations of heaviness and warmth in the limbs and an overall sense of rejuvenation or recuperation. Schultz worked to develop a technique that could achieve similar outcomes but relied on self-directed suggestions, thereby eliminating the dependence on a hypnotist or therapist. The conditions needed are the same as those for relaxation – comfortable sitting or lying position, quiet, loose clothing, and closed eyes.

Autogenic phrases may focus on suggestions for 'heaviness', suggestions for warmth, suggestions for regular heartbeat or regulation of breathing, or suggestions for cooling of the forehead. No matter what the desired effect, the phrases follow a certain structure. Below are examples of autogenic phrases adapted from the 1969 book by Luthe on *Autogenic Training*.

1. The content of the phrase should be directed at the desired outcome, for example, "My hands are warm."

2. Statements should be phrased positively, e.g., "My right hand is warm" rather than "My hands are not cold."

3. Modify any phrase that produces discomfort. For example, if the phrase "My arm is warm" produces discomfort, try "My arm is comfortable and relaxed" instead.

Emphasize a passive, nonjudgmental approach to the repetition of phrases. Have the patient start with a visual image of the part of the body toward which suggestions are directed, e.g., the hand, and a visual image of the autogenic phrase itself. Initially, each phrases should be repeated subvocally for 30 to 90 seconds. Phrases for heaviness can be used alone to reduce muscular tension, or in combination with EMG biofeedback. Phrases for warmth can be used alone or in combination with thermal biofeedback.

> **Phrases for comfort, heaviness, and warmth are commonly used for pain**

Guided Imagery

Imagery can be self-guided or therapist-guided. As with other forms of relaxation, audio recordings can be helpful both for learning and for maintaining

---

Clinical Pearl
Example of a Detailed Guided Imagery

Imagine you are standing on a beach and you take a step forward. As you do, the heel of your foot sinks into soft warm sand...the sand cups and molds around the heel of your foot. As you walk forward, the sand molds into the arch of your foot...around the ball of your foot and between your toes. The sand feels warm and soft...it molds around your footsteps. If you listen carefully, you can hear light crunching of the sand with each step. As you look out, you see bright white beach...trailing off as far as you can see. The sand is white...bright as diamonds gleaming in the sunlight. Off to your side is the ocean...stretching out...blue... until it meets the horizon. You see the waves roll in...the spray leaping up and glinting in the sun. The waves roll onto the beach...break...and glide back out. You hear the sound of the waves change...as they roll in...break...and glide back out. There is the constant, yet always changing, sound of the ocean. This sound is broken only by the sharp cry of sea gulls as they fly over the water...over the beach. The sun is high and bright. You feel it warm your skin. Your step feels strong and springy. You breathe in deeply and smell the salty air...the smell of the sea. Smells so invigorating...you pull your shoulders back and stand to your full height....your stride becomes longer...and stronger. You can walk as far and as long as you want...or you can sit or lay in the sand. You can watch the clouds... the waves...or you can lie back with your eyes closed...listening to the sounds and feeling the warm sun and the cool ocean breeze.

Clinical Pearl
Example of Unstructured Guided Imagery

Imagine being at the most beautiful place you can think of. It may be a place you have been before...or it may be a place you know only in your imagination. But it's beautiful...peaceful...and serene. Walk around...begin to see all the colors...notice the feel of the air on your skin...the smells. As you breathe in deeply, you drink in the fresh, scented air. It's quiet here. The sounds you hear are gentle, and add to the feeling of peacefulness. You can walk around...strolling slowly...soaking in the beauty of this place. You can sit or lie down. There are comfortable places to take in the beauty and serenity of this place.

practice. Patients often say that they find recorded practice helpful as it allows them to be recipients, and passively experience the relaxation/imagery, rather than having to be actively involved producing imagery. Therapist-guided imagery can involve images that are described at length and in great detail. Alternatively, the therapist can briefly present an image and then ask the patient to mentally fill in the details. The imagery should be introduced after the patient has slowed his or her breathing and developed a state of relaxation.

Images can be used to address pain more directly. The following can be helpful for patients who are having an exacerbation of pain and believe that they cannot redirect their attention away from the pain. As usual, the use of imagery begins after the patient is breathing slowly and regularly.

> Guided imagery can work well for patients who believe their mind is too active to allow them to relax

Clinical Pearl
Example of Guided Image to Change Pain

See yourself sitting in a chair...there's not much in the room around you...plain walls...a few simple pieces of furniture. Now as you sit, imagine holding your hands cupped in front of you. Now imagine your hands going to your pain and taking it out...take it right out of your body. Place your pain on the floor in front of you. As you watch it, it begins to take shape. It may take on a distinct shape... perhaps hard, with sharp edges...or it may be changing and without distinct edges...more like liquid or smoke. Your pain may have a color...it may be a bright and strong color...fiery red or orange...or it may light and indistinct...smoky blue-gray or airy yellow. Your pain may be large...or it may be small...but as you watch it, it becomes more and more clear. As you watch your pain, you can begin to make it change. You may find that you can change its color...or its shape...or its size. Whatever begins to happen is fine...let it happen. Let your pain begin to change... you may find that you can take the sharpness off of the edges...or the brightness out of the color. You may be able to change bright, hot red to pink. Let it begin to change...whether it's the form...the texture...the color...or the size. You may find that its becoming smaller and smaller. It may change a great deal...or just a little bit. Whatever happens is fine. Now reach down and take your pain back. Put it back where you got it...take a deep breath and slowly let your eyes open.

Hypnosis

Hypnosis was a primary vehicle for anesthesia during surgery until the mid-19th century

In 19th century India, a Scottish physician, James Esdaile, performed amputations and other surgical procedures with hypnosis as the sole method of pain control. He performed numerous surgeries, and his writings suggest that he obtained not only good control of pain with the use of hypnosis but also a decrease in mortality from such postsurgical complications as shock, infection, and hemorrhage. However, the introduction of nitrous oxide, ether and chloroform as more effective forms of anesthesia kept hypnosis from becoming widely used. Although used less than chemical anesthesia, hypnosis has since been used for surgery, childbirth, dental procedures, and burn debridement.

The phenomenon of hypnosis has been the subject of much debate. Various theories compete to explain hypnosis, the two most prominent being the dissociation theory and the sociocognitive theory. The dissociative theory suggests that cognitive control mechanisms become dissociated from each other in the hypnotic state, resulting in susceptibility to suggestion. The sociocognitive theory suggests that hypnosis is an interpersonal phenomenon in which the subject acts in response to social cues, expectations, and demand characteristics of the situation.

Three characteristics of hypnosis make it useful as a technique for managing pain:

- Physical relaxation.
- Openness to suggestion.
- Narrowing of the attentional field.

In the hypnotic state, attention narrows and becomes focused on the voice of the hypnotist. The subject is not asleep, under the control of the hypnotist, or in any way unconscious. In fact, the state of hypnosis could be described as one of heightened awareness.

It is not uncommon to experience hypnotic-like states during everyday events

In the hypnotic state, the subject becomes more open to suggestions given by the hypnotist. Hypnotic suggestibility is not equivalent to gullibility. What is required is curiosity, a willingness to suspend one's usual sense of reality, and to "see what happens" during hypnosis. This is similar to everyday occurrences such as watching a movie and suspending awareness of acting, sets, staged scenes, and scripted relationships to experience a different reality for a brief period of time. During hypnosis one can enter a state in which pain perceptions are temporarily altered.

Myths and misconceptions about hypnosis can impair a patient's ability to enter hypnosis

Many patients hold misconceptions about hypnosis, often based on stage shows and movie stereotypes. These beliefs can contribute to fears of being unduly controlled or of being made to engage in humiliating or otherwise unacceptable behaviors. It is essential for patients to be fully informed about the nature of hypnosis and have misunderstandings and misconceptions corrected before beginning. A patient must be allowed to either consent to or refuse hypnosis. Informing a patient about hypnosis should include, but not be limited to, the following points:

- During hypnosis, you will not be asleep or unconsciousness.
- Hypnosis is a state of heightened awareness; you will be aware of everything that happens to you.
- If you can be hypnotized, that does not mean that you are gullible, lacking intelligence, weak willed, or willing to let yourself be controlled.
- Being curious and willing to "see what happens" can make it easier for you to experience hypnosis.

There are many types of hypnotic inductions. No matter which one is used, several events should occur:

- The subject becomes quiet and relaxed.
- Attention is narrowed.
- An occurrence is linked to the suggestion of the hypnotist.

For example, the hypnotist can link his or her suggestion to an event such as eye closure. The patient is asked to focus his or her eyes at a point slightly above eye level. The induction begins with suggestions for comfort and relaxation and, as the induction progresses, for the eyes to become tired. The patient's eyes will naturally fatigue and begin to blink more rapidly, at which point the hypnotist may say, "As your eyes become more tired, you may find that you blink more often." As the eyelids begin to droop, the hypnotist says, "Your eyelids will become heavier and heavier," and eventually, "At some time, it will be more comfortable to let your eyes close than to keep them open. When that happens…just let your eyes close." In this way, the occurrence of the event, that is eye closure, becomes linked to the suggestion of the hypnotist.

Most hypnotic inductions include some type of preliminary instructions to facilitate eye closure followed by suggestions for relaxation. These suggestions are similar to those of a passive relaxation exercise and include suggestions for heaviness and comfort. As with other relaxation techniques, the patient should be in a comfortable position and distractions should be reduced or eliminated. During the induction and suggestions, the voice of the hypnotist should be soothing, with limited inflection; suggestions should be short, simple and repeated.

> Most hypnotic inductions include suggestions for relaxation and comfort

There are a number of techniques that can be used to alter pain perception or the response to pain. A few examples are below. Each of these techniques should be preceded by an induction. For further techniques see Roy Udolf's *Handbook of Hypnosis for Professionals* (1978).

Clinical Pearl
Examples of Hypnotic Suggestions for Pain Control

Pain dial (suggestions for altering pain intensity)

Your (painful limb or area of pain) sends signals to your brain. When those signals reach your brain, you experience pain. Because the brain is so complex many things can either "turn up" your pain or "turn down" your pain. Like using a dial on a radio or a thermostat, your pain can be turned up, or increased…or turned down, or decreased. I want to teach you how to use that dial to change your pain. Find an image of a dial or knob…it might be like a thermostat or radio dial… it doesn't matter what kind…but find a clear image of a dial. Now see if you can "turn up" your pain. It doesn't have to be a lot…just turn it up a little bit…let your pain increase. Now turn the dial in the other direction…turn it down a little bit… let your pain decrease. Up or down…when you want to…you can just leave the dial turned down.

Dissociation (suggestions for separating self from pain)

See yourself sitting in the chair…see how your hands fall…where your legs, your feet are…the position of your head. Now slowly begin to move back…imagine a camera filming a movie…the camera is on a dolly and moves back…farther back. You continue to see yourself but you appear more and more distant. You're looking at the person in the chair…you can see the person in the chair…but you move

Clinical Pearl (continued)

farther and farther away. You can watch the person in the chair from a different place in the room...from another chair...the top of the bookcase...or from high in the corner of the ceiling. You can float away and watch the person in the chair... you're free...and light...and can move around the room with great ease...light as a feather and able to float about to wherever you want to go. You can be aware of the person in the chair but you're light...floating...feeling free.

Neutralizing the pain experience (suggestions for decreasing the emotional response to pain)

Be aware of your pain...notice the feelings...the sensations. As you focus on the sensations, begin to describe them to yourself. Notice these feelings in detail...they may seem like shapeless feelings of hurt or pain but they are really very distinct sensations. They may be sharp...or burning...or aching. There may be feelings of pressure or twisting...or throbbing. Begin to describe to yourself the exact feelings. Notice how the feelings change...or how they're more intense at one place than in another. Is the feeling throbbing...tingling...sharp? Describe to yourself all of the changes you notice. You can be very aware of the feelings in your body...they are there, but they don't require any emotional response from you. You can feel them, describe them, but you don't have to be upset about them or do anything about them...just notice the feelings...then let them pass.

Obtain training to learn how to frame hypnotic suggestions and manage complications

Before using hypnosis with a patient, it is important to obtain some instruction. Hypnosis rarely produces any serious adverse effects although most of the problems that do occur are due to the inexperience of the hypnotist. Instruction can be obtained by attending training workshops and or working with an experienced hypnotist to learn the techniques and skills of hypnosis. During hypnosis, subjects respond to suggestions in a concrete or literal manner, and learning how to frame suggestions is an essential part of hypnotic technique. It is important to learn how to manage complications, such as when a subject does not come out of trance on cue, and how to frame suggestions for self-hypnosis and posthypnotic suggestions

Biofeedback

Biofeedback provides information about physiologicial functions

Biofeedback devices enable patients to become aware of, and thereby to develop conscious control over, bodily processes of which they are usually unaware and that are usually not under conscious control. They provide immediate auditory and/or visual feedback about fluctuations in a specific physical parameter such as whether the level of tension in a particular muscle is increasing or decreasing. The two most common modalities used for the treatment of chronic pain are electromyographic and thermal biofeedback.

Electromyograhic biofeedback is used to treat non-migraine headaches and soft tissue injuries

Electromyograhphic (EMG) biofeedback is used to help patients learn to decrease muscle tension in tension headaches and in pain disorders with a significant muscle tension component such as soft tissue injuries. The patient is seated comfortably and sensors are placed at specific muscle sites. The placement sites depend on the particular muscles that are contributing to the pain problem. The monitor detects minute changes in electrical activity at the lead sites, amplifies these signals, and displays them in a visual or auditory form. The patient uses this feedback to learn positions, postures, and techniques

---

Clinical Pearl
Developing Sensations of Warmth

Examples of autogenic phrases for hand warming:
> My hands and arms feel warm and heavy.
> My hands are warm, relaxed, and comfortable.
> Warmth is flowing into my hands...into my fingertips.
> My hands are warm, heavy, and relaxed.

Examples of images for warmth:
> Image of a beach scene.
> Wrapping the hands around a warm coffee mug.
> Holding the hands outstretched in front of a fireplace.
> Placing the hands in a basin of hot water.

---

that decrease the tension in the monitored muscles. Relaxation techniques, diaphragmatic breathing, autogenic phrases, meditation, and imagery can be incorporated into biofeedback training.

Thermal biofeedback is used with migraine headaches, reflex sympathetic dystrophy (RSD), and Reynaud's disease. The temperature sensor used in thermal biofeedback is called a thermistor. It is usually placed at the tip of the patient's index finger. The biofeedback monitor provides visual or auditory information in real time about temperature fluctuations. With the aid of this feedback, patients can to learn to warm their hands and raise their peripheral temperature. For migraine headaches, vasodilation is thought to be the mechanism of treatment. In reflex sympathetic dystrophy and Reynaud's disease, increased blood flow, and warming of the affected limb are thought to provide relief. Patients can use various techniques to induce peripheral warming, including relaxation, autogenic phrases, and imagery.

Thermal biofeedback is used in the treatment of migraine headache, RSD, and Reynaud's disease

With all forms of biofeedback, home practice of relaxation, imagery, and/or autogenic phrases is essential for incorporating the skills into everyday life. Patients should be instructed to practice for at least 20 minutes each day.

For the practitioner, it is important to obtain the skills needed to use biofeedback effectively with patients. Learning about the instrumentation, how to introduce biofeedback to patients, suggestions for sequences of sessions, placement of leads, techniques for relaxation of muscle tension and for hand-warming, suggestions for cued practice, and dealing with complications can be obtained from texts such as that by Schwartz and Andrasik (2003), workshops, and/or from experienced practitioners of biofeedback.

4.4 Efficacy and Prognosis

Evaluation of the efficacy of cognitive-behavioral therapy for chronic pain is plagued by several difficulties. First, studies vary in how successful treatment outcome is defined making it difficult to generalize results across studies. Some of the most common definitions include: pain reduction, pain interfer-

CBT has been found to be effective with a variety of chronic pain conditions

ence (the extent to which pain interferes with daily activity), improved mood, fewer pain behaviors, decreased use of pain medications, return to work, and decreased health care utilization. Second, while participating in psychological intervention trials, many patients are taking prescription medications and may be undergoing medical procedures or attending physical therapy. This makes it difficult to ascertain which treatment or combination of treatments influences the selected outcome variables. Third, there is a lack of uniformity across cognitive-behavioral programs. In 1999, Morley, Eccelston, and Williams conducted a meta-analysis of 25 studies across a variety of pain conditions. All of these studies included some type of psychological intervention such as bio-feedback, relaxation, behavioral therapy, or cognitive-behavioral therapy, but there was little consistency among studies as to which elements were included. Patients in some of the studies also attended physical therapy or occupational therapy, while other were undergoing concurrent medical treatments. Thus, outcome studies are often complicated by nonstudy treatments, and generaliz-ability of the results is influenced by the lack of consistency in treatment components and outcome variables. Despite these difficulties, cognitive-behavioral therapy for chronic pain has demonstrated positive outcomes in a number of studies. Outcome studies have been done with specific conditions, primarily low back pain, and with heterogeneous pain conditions.

CBT has been found to be effective with chronic low back pain (Guzman, Esmail, Karjalainen, Malmivaara, Irvin, & Bombardier, 2001; Hoffman, Chat-koff, Papas, & Kerns, 2007; Ostelo, Van Tulder, Vlaeyan, Linton, Morley, & Assendelft, 2005; Van Tulder, Ostelo, Vlaeyen, Linton, Morley, & Assendelft, 2000). The meta-analysis by Hoffman et al. (2007), reviewed 22 RCTs compar-ing outpatient psychological interventions (individual and multidisciplinary) with control groups (wait-list and treatment as usual). When psychological interventions (individual and multidisciplinary) were collapsed and compared to all control conditions (wait-list and treatment as usual), psychological in-terventions were found to be superior to control conditions. On treatment out-come variables of pain intensity and pain-related interference, all psychologi-cal interventions were superior to wait-list, but not active, control conditions posttreatment. CBT demonstrated superiority in reducing posttreatment pain intensity when compared to wait-list controls. Self-regulatory treatments such as relaxation and biofeedback demonstrated superiority to wait-list controls at reducing pain intensity and depression posttreatment. As with other stud-ies, (Ostelo et al., 2005; van Tulder et al., 2000), psychological intervention provided no significant benefit over active control conditions. In the Hoffman review, there was however, one exception. Multidisciplinary programs were found to be superior to active controls in improving return to work outcomes at short-term and long-term follow-up. Guzman et al. (2001) also found CBT programs to be effective in reducing pain and improving function when com-pared to treatment as usual for low back pain although efficacy was related to program intensity with longer time and more contact demonstrating the superior treatment.

Similar results were found in reviews of psychological interventions for arthritis pain and heterogeneous pain conditions. The APA Division 12 Task Force on Psychological Interventions found CBT to be an empirically sup-ported therapy based largely on Keefe and colleagues' (1990a, b) studies of

CBT for arthritic knee pain and Parker and colleagues' (1988) trial of CBT for rheumatoid arthritis pain (Chambless et al., 1998). In their 1999 review and meta-analysis, Morley et al. concluded that cognitive-behavioral interventions (including biofeedback and operant therapy) were effective in the treatment of various pain conditions in comparison to wait list controls. When compared to wait-list controls, CBT was superior in the domains of pain experience, mood/affect, reducing negative coping and increasing positive coping, increasing activity level, and social role function. When compared to active controls, CBT retained efficacy as a treatment although in fewer domains (pain experience, positive coping, and social role function).

In 1995, the National Institutes of Health (NIH) issued a Technology Assessment Conference Statement regarding the use of behavioral and relaxation approaches in the treatment of chronic pain and insomnia. The participants included a 12-member review panel and 23 experts representing the fields of family medicine, psychiatry, psychology, public health, nursing, pain medicine, sleep medicine, behavioral medicine, neurology, and the neurosciences. The review panel concluded that there is strong evidence for the effectiveness of relaxation in reducing chronic pain associated with various medical conditions, and strong evidence for the use of hypnosis for alleviating cancer pain. There is moderate evidence that hypnosis is effective for use in other chronic pain conditions such as irritable bowel syndrome, oral mucositis, temporomandibular disorder, and tension headaches, and moderate evidence that cognitive behavioral therapies are efficacious in alleviating chronic pain.

Overall, there is consistent and respectable evidence that CBT is effective as a treatment for chronic pain. CBT has most often demonstrated efficacy when compared to wait-list controls although it has also shown efficacy when compared to active controls on some outcome variables. The definition of psychological interventions ranges from single modality approaches, e.g., relaxation or operant therapy, to multimodal approaches, e.g., cognitive–behavioral treatment in the broadest sense of the term, to multidisciplinary therapies which include medical treatment and/or physical therapy in addition to psychological therapies and each treatment approach shows some efficacy on different outcome measures. There is less evidence for individual components of CBT, although relaxation, biofeedback, hypnosis, and cognitive therapy have demonstrated treatment efficacy as independent treatments. Some components, such as imagery and distraction, have been adapted from acute pain treatment where efficacy has been demonstrated. Other elements of CBT either have not been studied independent of a CBT program or have not demonstrated treatment efficacy independent of a CBT or multidisciplinary program. The question remains as to what "mix" of components will be the most effective on which outcome variables for which individual.

4.5   Mechanisms of Action

The above-mentioned 1995 NIH Technology Assessment Conference Statement reviewed the candidate mechanisms of action that had been proposed for relaxation, hypnosis, and cognitive behavior therapy. Several different mechanisms

There are multiple suggested mechanisms of action for psychological interventions

of action were suggested for relaxation techniques including altered sympathetic activity (reduction in respiration rate, basal heart rate, and metabolism) enhanced parasympathetic activity and, in some reports, increased EEG slow wave activity.

In a RCT by Turner, Holtzman, and Mancl (2007), patients with temporomandibular disorder (TMD) who received CBT versus an educational/attention control group demonstrated significantly greater improvement at one-year follow-up on activity interference, pain intensity, and disability. This study assessed variables that mediated the effects of CBT on TMD pain and disability at one year and found the primary mediating variables entailed changes in pain-related beliefs. The primary mediating variables were: an increase in the perceived ability to control pain and self-efficacy for managing TMD pain, decrease in beliefs that pain is disabling, that pain signals harm and in catastrophizing.

Activation of selected cortical areas has been associated with reductions in pain unpleasantness and pain intensity. These findings suggest that pain is a heterogeneous experience, and that there exists no single center for the experience of pain in the central nervous system. For example, hypnotic suggestions have been associated with a distinctive pattern of brain activity (Rainville, Duncan, Price, Carrier, & Bushnell, 1997; Rainville, Hofbauer, Tomas, Duncan, Bushnell, & Price, 1999) in which hypnotic suggestions for reduction in pain unpleasantness selectively activated cortical areas associated with emotion, but not areas involved in pain sensation. However, hypnotic suggestions to decrease pain intensity were paralleled by a decrease in pain unpleasantness. These studies suggest that the limbic structures of the brain are associated with the emotional aspects of pain while the somatosensory areas are associated with the sensory aspects of pain.

In two studies looking at the effect of distraction using fMRI (Tracey et al., 2002; Valet et al., 2004), activation in the periaqueductal gray (PAG) area of the brain was significantly increased during distraction conditions. The increase in activation predicted changes in perceived pain intensity suggesting that the PAG can inhibit pain signal transmission. A possible mechanism for this decreased pain intensity during the distraction condition is the release of endogenous opioids with activation of the PAG. The relationship between biological and psychological phenomena suggests that understanding the mechanism of action depends on both the treatment and the level of the system being investigated.

4.6   Variations and Combinations of Methods

Treatment of chronic pain is most often multidisplinary and/ or multimodal due to its complexity

Multidisciplinary care is the most effective way to treat chronic pain. No single therapy provides adequate relief in most cases of chronic pain. A specific, individualized combination of therapies should be chosen to meet the patient's unique needs. In addition to the treatments discussed above, physical therapy and various complementary and alternative therapies are often used for the treatment of chronic pain. For the therapeutic approaches listed below, seek out an experienced practitioner to whom you can refer patients.

4.6.1 Physical Therapy

For many, if not most, individuals who suffer with chronic pain, activity and exercise worsen pain. However, lack of exercise can also worsen pain over time through deconditioning. Physical inactivity can cause significant loss of muscle tone, and as the muscles become deconditioned, exercise (and even movement) becomes increasingly painful. Deconditioning also affects cardio-vascular fitness such that the heart works less efficiently, leading to fatigue and decreased endurance. Exercise and conditioning programs must be tailored to the needs of the individual and should be lead by a knowledgeable physical therapist. An exercise regimen should be implemented with the goals of improving strength, flexibility, and endurance without exacerbating pain. This is not to imply that exercise will never be painful, but patients must learn to distinguish "good pain," i.e., harmless pain associated with building muscle, from "bad pain" or exercise that seriously exacerbates the underlying painful condition. Graduated exercise protocols can help patients increase their exercise tolerance and fitness with minimal exacerbation of pain. Exercise can help strengthen and stabilize muscles around the spine and painful joints. It can also improve sleep and energy, and help with weight loss. Weight loss can, in turn, reduce stress and strain on painful joints.

> **A combination of treatments provides better pain relief and broadens the repertoire of pain coping skills**

> **Lack of movement and exercise can increase pain and decrease endurance**

Many physical therapists are skilled in instructing patients on the use of transcutaneous electrical nerve stimulation or TENS units. TENS units use pulses of electricity to stimulate painful areas. They are small enough to be worn on a belt and are programmable. TENS is thought to relieve pain by stimulating myelinated nerve fibers which, in turn, inhibits the transmission of pain signals along unmyelinated C fibers.

4.6.2 Complementary and Alternative Medicine (CAM)

Complementary and alternative therapies include products and practices that are not considered part of conventional medical treatment. Most CAM therapies lack rigorous scientific evidence regarding their safety and effectiveness for various medical conditions. If rigorous research ever does show that a particular CAM therapy is safe and efficacious, it may leave the CAM domain and enter mainstream medical practice.

> **As the evidence base for CAM therapies increases, some therapies become mainstream medicine**

Complementary treatments are used in conjunction with traditional medical treatments whereas alternative treatments are used in place of conventional medical therapies. The National Center for Complementary and Alternative Medicine, one of the National Institutes of Health, classifies five categories of CAM therapies:

1. *Alternative medical or healing systems.* These include homeopathic and naturopathic systems in the United States, and many non-Western systems such as traditional Chinese medicine.
2. *Mind-body connections.* Some of these therapies, such as hypnosis, relaxation, biofeedback, and meditation have become mainstream therapies. The underlying concept of the mind-body connection is that the mind has some ability to influence physical functions.
3. *Herbs and dietary supplements* include herbs, food, and vitamins that

are considered to be "natural" or found in nature rather than manufactured.

4. *Manipulation therapies* include techniques that involve touch and/or manipulations of part of the body such as massage and chiropractic treatment.

5. *Energy therapies* are based on the belief that the flow of energy in the body can become unbalanced. The therapy is designed to rebalance the energy flow and include such techniques as acupuncture, Reiki, and magnet therapy.

Acupuncture and massage are often used for chronic pain, either as complementary or alternative treatments. There is growing evidence that some of these therapies may help to relieve chronic pain.

Acupuncture is based on the ancient Chinese medical concept that diseases are due to imbalances in the body's flow of energy. More than 2000 acupuncture points connect the pathways along which bodily energy or "qi" is believed to flow. Needles inserted in these points release blocked energy flow, thus restoring balance. Within the framework of Western medicine, there is limited understanding of how acupuncture works. Several hypotheses have been considered, including the release of biochemicals such as endorphins, neurotransmitters, and neurohormones.

Massage therapy:

- *Sports massage* focuses on muscles relevant to the sporting activity. It is used to decrease the chances of injury and speed recovery following injury.
- *Shiatsu and traditional Thai massage* use pressure on the body's "energy points" and "energy lines."
- *Trigger point or pressure point massage* focuses on trigger points, or small muscle spasms, that can develop following damage to a muscle.
- *Swedish massage* is used to relax muscles by applying pressure to them. It also has other aims, such as to improve circulation, stimulate the skin, and increase the suppleness of tendons and ligaments.

> **Acupuncture and massage therapy have shown some efficacy with various pain disorders**

4.7 Problems in Carrying Out the Treatments

Reliance on the Medical Model

> **One barrier to treatment is a lack of knowledge about the complexity of chronic pain and treatment**

One of the barriers to implementation of psychological treatment of chronic pain is the exclusive reliance on the medical model in many settings. Many medical schools provide only limited training in the treatment of pain. Both providers and patients are often unaware of the psychological complexity of pain or of the role that multidisciplinary therapies can play in its treatment. Fortunately, medical schools are beginning to introduce courses specifically designed to address the understanding, and treatment, of pain.

Patient Comprehension

Patients may have little understanding about what is causing their pain and hold misconceptions about doing further damage or about an underlying disease process. Physical therapy or any increase in activity can result in increased pain, and patients must learn to distinguish pain resulting from mobilizing deconditioned muscles from baseline pain. Patients should be informed about the nature of chronic pain in general, their pain in particular, and of the relevance of the proposed treatments.

Commitment of Time and Effort

A significant barrier to patient adherence to psychological therapies is the level of commitment and degree of motivation required to learn and practice time-consuming therapies. Psychological interventions often require changes in daily habits and interpersonal interactions. Implementing lifestyle changes such as pacing and modifying activities, improving patterns of communication, and following an exercise regimen requires a high level of personal commitment and motivation. Learning relaxation, hypnosis, meditation, or biofeedback generally requires at least 8 to 12 one-hour sessions plus home practice. Such changes are daunting even under normal circumstances, but when added to the fatigue, physical limitations, and emotional consequences of pain, they can present exceptional challenges. Because it can be difficult to sustain motivation to adhere to treatment recommendations, some type of ongoing support is often needed. Potential sources of this support include community-based chronic pain support groups, therapist-led support groups, and individual follow-up sessions.

Maintaining motivation can be a barrier to the practice of psychological interventions

Therapist Barriers

Undertaking therapy with patients suffering with chronic pain can be challenging. The combination of demoralization, physical deconditioning, anger, and skepticism toward new treatment approaches (particularly psychological interventions) can leave therapists feeling frustrated and ineffectual. Patients referred for psychological intervention, whether for individual or group treatment, are rarely self-referred and often have little understanding about how a psychologist can be helpful in the treatment of their pain. It is important not to be drawn into the belief that if the person's pain would be adequately treated or cured, their psychosocial difficulties would disappear. Although this may (or may not) be true, for patients with chronic pain it is not an option. Patients will present pain as the reason they cannot complete assignments. A patient may say that he or she did not start a walking program, or go to lunch with a friend, or get out of the house three times in a week because of pain. It is important to evaluate the proposed assignment with the patient in order to determine whether the task is too difficult and should be broken into simpler steps, or whether fears or habits are contributing to nonadherence.

4.8   Multicultural Issues

Despite many advances in the field of pain management, pain is still undertreated, particularly among ethnic and racial minority groups. In 1999, an Institute of Medicine Study Committee was formed to assess factors that contributed to disparities in the delivery of health care services to minorities and to recommend interventions to address them. Disparities based on race, age, and

Disparities in treatment have been found across disease entities and treatment settings

gender were found across disease entities and treatment settings. Factors within two major areas were considered as the primary contributors to racial and ethnic disparities: (a) problems within the health care systems, such as access to treatment and (b) patient-provider factors which included discrimination based on biases, stereotyping, and problems with communication. Specific barriers to adequate treatment of pain include communication problems between patients and providers, concerns about risks of addiction, abuse and diversion of opioid analgesics, and lack of training for health care professionals in the treatment of pain. Disparities in treatment can be influenced by problems in communication. Ethnic differences in expectations about the inevitability of pain, fears of addiction to potent analgesics, and varying degrees of education about appropriate management of pain influence treatment. Racial and ethnic minority patients reported less involvement in medical decision-making, although recent studies have indicated that patients are more actively involved in their own care when their physicians are of the same ethnic background. Physician decisions about treatment for painful conditions are open to influence by factors such as patient characteristics, practice setting, and the social context due to limited established guidelines for treatment of a range of painful conditions.

Various factors can influence disparities in treatment

A review by Green and colleagues (2003) found ethnic and racial disparities in the treatment of pain across types of pain and in all settings such as emergency departments and for postoperative pain. Several studies have shown disparities in the use of analgesics with minority patients in both inpatient and outpatient settings. For patients seen in emergency department settings, Hispanics and Blacks received fewer analgesic medications compared to non-Hispanic Whites, even when injuries and pain ratings were comparable. These disparities continue into postoperative settings as suggested in a study by Ng, Dimsdale, Shragg, and Deutsch (1996). They found that White, Black, and Hispanic patients being treated for pain following similar operative procedures were administered different doses of analgesics: Whites received the highest dosages; Hispanics received about half as much.

Racial and ethnic disparities in the use of analgesics for pain were found in ED and postoperative settings

4.9   Conclusion

The treatment of patients with chronic pain can be a challenging, yet rewarding, process. Patients often come in tired, angry, deconditioned, demoralized, and apathetic, having lost much of what was of value in their lives. Across disciplines, there are a variety of treatment approaches that can help patients manage their pain. Yet even with comprehensive, multidisciplinary treatment, at best what we have to offer is reduction of symptoms and improvement in functioning. It can be difficult for both patients and health care professionals to accept a less than totally satisfying solution to a problem. But, as we remind our patients, progress must be measured by whatever small successes we can achieve. Many patients come to our clinic with the idea that pain management is the "end of the road." However, with patience, education, a willingness to hear about the impact of pain on their lives, and to understand the daily struggle of coping with pain, helping patients manage pain can, instead, be the first steps on a new road.

5

Case Vignette

Mr. J. is a 52-year-old married, white male who developed back pain following a fall at work, which ruptured a disk. He underwent lumbar spine surgery but continues to experience aching and grinding pain in his low back with burning pain radiating into his right leg. During the two years since his surgery, he has been unable to work at his job as a construction worker, has settled his claim with the company for which he worked, and is presently receiving social security disability payments.

Mr. J. has been tried on numerous pain medications and is currently prescribed Darvocet, two per day, and Neurontin 300 mg three times a day. He reports that his medications "help a little bit" when he is inactive and sitting in his recliner. He states that he sometimes takes extra Darvocet when he is more active, for example, while on vacation with his family. He has run out of Darvocet several times and says that his family physician will no longer prescribe pain medications because he increased his use of opioid analgesics. He has had no injection therapies but has attended physical therapy, consisting primarily of passive modalities, and he states that they provided only modest relief. Exercises increase his pain. He has no home exercise program or general conditioning regimen. He rates his pain as between a 6/10 and a 9/10, increasing when he is more active and decreasing with rest. A hot shower provides some modest relief.

Mr. J. spends his days watching TV and "puttering" in the garage where he used to enjoy working on cars as a hobby. His wife has returned to work because of the financial difficulties they have experienced since his unemployment. She attended the initial evaluation and expressed anger and resentment about having had to take over responsibility for managing the household, both financially and physically. She works, cares for the household and yard, and feels overwhelmed. She believes that her husband can do more than he presently does and that he has "gotten lazy" since he has been unemployed. He says that he tries to help, but because doing house or yard work worsens his pain, he has stopped trying.

During the evaluation, Mr. J. sat toward the edge of his chair, shifted his posture frequently, and directed his gaze toward the floor. He presents as a modestly obese man whose grooming is somewhat negligent; he has several days' growth of beard, and his torn shirttail is untucked and unbuttoned. His affect is sad. He describes himself as "frustrated" and "worthless" because he can no longer do what he did in the past. His wife believes that he has been depressed since being unable to return to work. Due to pain, he is no longer involved with activities he previously enjoyed such as working on cars and bowling, although he believes he would still enjoy doing these things if he were able. He no longer visits with family, sees his bowling buddies, or goes to the movies with his wife, saying he "would just rather stay home." He is "tired of explaining that [he's] not better" and believes that "people think [he's] faking because [he] looks OK." He describes his sleep as poor, stating that he stays up and watches TV until he is tired, then sleeps in two-hour stretches, getting up to smoke a cigarette or watch TV. He is "up and down" all night and believes that he averages 3–4 hours of sleep a night. He denies napping during the day, but his wife says that he nods off while watching TV. He states that he is rarely hungry, although he snacks or eats quick foods throughout the day. He "picks at" dinner, which his wife prepares. Despite decreased appetite, he reported a forty-pound weight gain, which he believes to be attributable to change in activity. He describes his short-term memory as "terrible," stating that he forgets appointments and chores his wife asks him to do during the day. He reports being unable to concentrate like he did in the past, but that he "doesn't have much to concentrate on anyway." He denies frank suicidal thoughts, plans, or intent, although he "doesn't know how long [he] can go on like this." He denied psychiatric history in himself or family of origin, and he has not been prescribed an antidepressant with the exception of amitriptyline 25 mg to help with sleep.

Mr. J. is the third eldest of six children. His parents are both deceased and he has little contact with his siblings. He completed high school, began working with his father in construction and worked at this profession until his injury. He resides with his wife of 30 years; they have two children who are married and live independently. Mr. J. smokes 1–1½ packs of cigarettes per day, and has smoked for over thirty years. He denied current use of alcohol, although he reports a history of alcohol abuse (1–2 six-packs of beer nightly, with two DUIs) dating back twenty-five years. He denied use of illicit drugs.

Considerations for Treatment Planning

- Medical treatment has been minimal.
  - He has had no injection therapies, is prescribed limited opioids analgesics and has had an inadequate trial of Neurontin.
  - He has some risk factors for developing addiction, such as a past history of alcohol abuse and unsanctioned dose increases of his opioid analgesics. However, his alcohol abuse history is remote and the opioid dose increases appear to be limited to times when he tries to be more active. Consider pseudoaddiciton, i.e., inadequately treated pain, as the reason for his increasing use of pain medications.
  - Mr. J. should be considered for spinal cord stimulation if conservative treatment does not provide relief.
- Physical therapies have been inadequate and Mr. J. is clearly deconditioned.
  - His physical therapy to date has consisted primarily of passive modalities.
  - What exercise therapy he has had resulted in increased pain, and he now engages in no home exercise program or conditioning exercise.

- The impact of pain on Mr. J.'s life has been significant.
  - He is no longer employed and this has affected his family's income, his self-image, his relationship with his wife, and his daily routine.
  - His recreational activities were also physically demanding. He no longer engages in activities he enjoyed, which limits his social contact.
  - He presents with symptoms of depression including sad affect, social withdrawal, feelings of worthlessness, disrupted nonrestorative sleep, diminished appetite, and impaired memory and concentration. He denies frank suicidal thoughts, plans, or intent, although he presents some future risk as he "doesn't know how long [he] can go on like this." He has been prescribed amitriptyline 25 mg for sleep, which is clearly ineffective for his sleep disturbance, and too small of a dose to be efficacious for depression.

Treatment Plan

- Contact his family physician and recommend referral to a pain management specialist for consideration of injection therapies and for medication consultation.
- Request orders from the referring physician for physical therapy with a therapist trained in treatment of chronic pain. Mr. J. may benefit from instruction in individualized exercises but most certainly requires instruction in a slowly progressing conditioning program. He may benefit from a trial of a TENS unit.
- Discuss with his referring or family physician the addition of an antidepressant, such as a SSRI to treat depression, and either increasing amitriptyline or changing to trazodone to help with sleep and decrease risk of further weight gain.
- Provide education about chronic pain for Mr. J. and his wife and have several sessions with them to identify and resolve problems that have developed in their marriage secondary to his pain and physical limitations.
- Assist Mr. J. with developing better sleep hygiene.
- Develop long- and short-term goals for meaningful daily activity and socialization. Refer for vocational rehabilitation if he expresses interest in retraining.
- Assist Mr. J. with developing structure for his days and ways to slowly increase and pace his daytime activity.
- Develop techniques for self-management of pain such as relaxation and meditation.
- Assist Mr. J. with smoking cessation or recommend programs such as those available through local hospitals or the American Lung Association.
- Treat depression by identifying and restructuring negative pain-related thoughts, beliefs, and expectations.

DSM-IV Diagnoses

Axis I: 311.0 Depression NOS
           305.10 Nicotine Dependence
           305.00 Alcohol Abuse, full remission
Axis II: No Diagnosis
Axis III: Chronic low back and right lower extremity pain
           (Consider this as the primary diagnosis if you use health and behavior codes.)

6

Further Reading

Patient-Focused Handbooks and Workbooks

These books are divided into chapters that focus on pain-related problem with techniques and suggestions for self-management. Many have logs, patient diaries, and homework to help incorporate techniques and lifestyle adjustments.

Caudill, M. (2001). *Managing pain before it manages you* (revised edition). New York: Guilford Press.
  Excellent homework examples.
Jamison, R. N. (1996). *Learning to master your chronic pain*. Sarasota, FL: Professional Resource Press.
  A companion manual is available for the professional that includes chapters on assessment, report-writing, and how to develop a cognitive behavioral group program.
Nicholas, M., Molloy, A., Tonkin, L., & Beeston, L. (2002). *Manage your pain*. Sydney: Australian Broadcasting Corporation.
  Additional chapters provide information about medical treatments and physical therapy exercises and conditioning.
Turk, D. C., & Winter, F. (2005). *The pain survival guide: How to reclaim your life*. Washington, DC: American Psychological Association.
  Excellent resources for additional reading and for research supporting cognitive-behavioral therapy for chronic pain.

Practitioner-Focused Books

These books cover a broad range of topics including the evolution of pain theories, psychological techniques and strategies for the management of pain, addressing family issues, depression, anxiety, exercise, and motivation.

Gatchel, R. J. (2005). *Clinical essentials of pain management*. Washington, DC: American Psychological Association.
Gatchel, R. J., & Turk, D. C. (Eds.) (1996). *Psychological approaches to pain management: A practitioner's handbook*. New York: Guilford Press.
Hadjistavropoulos, T., & Craig, K. D. (Eds.) (2004). *Pain: Psychological perspectives*. Mahwah, NJ: Lawrence Erlbaum.
  Comprehensive coverage of the psychology of pain from the evolution of pain theories, cultural and social contexts, pain across the life span assessment, and psychological interventions for acute and chronic pain. Each chapter reviews evidence for the theories and treatment practices presented.

Cognitive Therapy for Chronic Pain

Thorn, B. E. (2004). *Cognitive therapy for chronic pain: A step-by-step guide*. New York: Guilford Press.
  This book is a detailed guide to the cognitive elements of therapy for chronic pain. The heart of the book includes detailed examples of session objectives, ways to work

through negative and distorted thoughts and beliefs, examples of patient-therapist dialogues, and homework assignments through ten treatment modules.

Assessment

Turk, D. C., & Melzack, R. (Eds.) (2001). *Handbook of Pain Assessment* (2nd ed.). New York: Guilford Press.
The most comprehensive book on the measurement of pain and assessment of people with pain. Sections include pain assessment and measures, the behavioral expression of pain, assessment of function and disability, psychological evaluation, and assessment of specific pain states. Excellent resource for developing a battery of measures for psychological evaluation.

Presurgical Psychological Screening

Block, A. R. (1996). *Presurgical psychological screening in chronic pain syndromes: A guide for the behavioral health practitioner.* Mahwah, NJ: Lawrence Erlbaum.
Block's book provides guidelines for presurgical psychological screening and the selection process for determining patient readiness for surgery based on psychosocial risk factors.

Hypnosis

Practical suggestions for developing hypnotic states and using hypnotic suggestions for pain management.
Kirsch, I., Capafons, A., Cardena-Buelna, E., & Amigo, S. (1999). *Clinical hypnosis and self-regulation: Cognitive-behavioral perspectives.* Washington, DC: American Psychological Association.
Udolf, R. (1987). *Handbook of hypnosis for professionals.* New York: Van Nostrand Reinhold.

Relaxation and Meditation

Benson, H. (1976). *The relaxation response.* New York: William Morrow.
Kabat-Zinn, J. (1990). *Full catastrophe living.* New York: Delta Books.
Young, S. (2004). *Break through pain: A step-by-step mindfulness meditation program for transforming chronic and acute pain.* Boulder, CO: Sound True, Inc.

Communication

Pachter, B. (2000). *The power of positive confrontation: The skills you need to know to handle conflicts at work, home and in life.* New York: Marlowe & Co.
Excellent techniques for developing communication skills in difficult situations that are simple and direct and which strive to decrease defensive and angry responses from others.

Biofeedback

Schwartz, M. S., & Andrasik, F. (2003). *Biofeedback: A practitioner's guide* (3rd ed.). New York: Guilford Press.
The most comprehensive text on biofeedback.

Websites

http://www.painfoundation.org/
http://www.ampainsoc.org/
http://www.nationalpainfoundation.org/

References

American Medical Association. (2007). *Current Procedural Terminology*. Chicago: Author.

American Psychiatric Association. (2000). *Diagnostic and statistical manual of mental disorders* (4th ed., text rev.). Washington, DC: American Psychiatric Association.

Andersson, G. B. (1999). Epidemiological features of chronic low back pain. *Lancet, 351,* 581–585.

Banks, S. M., & Kerns, R. D. (1996). Explaining high rates of depression in chronic pain: A diathesis-stress framework. *Psychological Bulletin, 119,* 95–110.

Beck, A. T. (1976). *Cognitive therapy and the emotional disorders*. New York: International Universities Press.

Beck, A. T., Steer, R. A., & Brown, B. K. (1996). Beck Depression Inventory Manual (2nd ed.). San Antonia, TX: Psychological Corporation.

Bellamy, N., Campbell, J., Robinson, V., Gee, T., Bourne, R., & Wells, G. (2006). Intraarticular corticosteroid for treatment of osteoarthritis of the knee. *The Cochrane Database of Systematic Reviews,* Art. No.: CD005328.

Bergner, M., Bobbitt, R. A., Carter, W. B., & Gibson, B. S. (1981). The Sickness Impact Profile: Development and final revision of a health status measure. *Medical Care, 19,* 787–805.

Block, A. (1996). Presurgical psychological screening in chronic pain syndromes: *Guide for the behavioral health practitioner*. Mahwah, NJ: Lawrence Erlbaum Associates.

Burchiel, K. J., Anderson, V. C., Wilson, B. J., Denison, D. B., Olson, K. A., & Shatin, D. (1995). Prognostic factors of spinal cord stimulation for chronic back and leg pain. *Neurosurgery, 36,* 1101–1111.

Burckhardt, C. S., Goldenberg, D., Crofford, L., Gerwin, R., Gowans, S., Jackson, K., et al. (2005). *Guideline for the management of fibromyalgia syndrome pain in adults and children*. APS Clinical Practice Guidelines Series, No. 4. Glenview, IL: American Pain Society.

Chambless, D. L., Baker, M. J., Baucom, D. H., Beutler, L. E., Calhoun, K. S., Crits-Christoph, P. et al. (1998). Update on empirically validated therapies, II. *The Clinical Psychologist, 51,* 3–16.

Chui, Y. H., Silman, A. J., Macfarlane, D. R., Gupta, A., Dickens, C., Morriss, R., & McBeth, J. (2005). Poor sleep and depression are independently associated with reduced pain threshold: results of a population based study. *Pain, 115,* 316–321.

Cook, R. J., & Sackett, D. L. (1995). The number needed to treat: A clinically useful measure of treatment effect. *BMJ, 310,* 452–454.

Cousins, M. J., & Bridenbaugh, P. O. (Eds.). (1998). *Neural blockade in clinical anesthesia and management of pain*. (3rd ed.) Philadelphia: Lippincott-Raven.

DeBruin, A. F., Diederiks, J. P. M., DeWitte, L. P., Stevens, L. P., & Philipsen, H. (1994). Assessing the responsiveness of a functional status measure: The Sickness Impact Profile versus the SIP68. *Journal of Clinical Epidemiology, 50,* 529–540.

Deyo, R. A., & Weinstein, J. N. (2001). Low Back Pain. *New England Journal of Medicine, 344,* 363–370.

Dunbar, S. A., & Katz, N. P. (1996). Chronic opioid therapy for nonmalignant pain in patients with a history of substance abuse: Report of 20 cases. *Journal of Pain and Symptom Management, 11,* 163–71.

Engel, G. L. (1977). The need for a new medical model. *Science, 196,* 129–136.

Fairbank, J. C., Couper, J., Davies, J. B., & O'Brien, J. P. (1980). The Oswestry low back pain questionnaire. *Physiotherapy*, *66*, 271–273.

Fishbain, D. A., Goldberg, M., Rosomoff, R. S., & Rosomoff, H. (1991). Case Reports: Completed suicide in chronic pain. *Clinical Journal of Pain*, *7*, 29–37.

Fishbain, D. A., Cutler, R., Rosomoff, H. L., & Rosomoff, R. S. (1997). Chronic pain associated depression: Antecedent or consequence of chronic pain? A review. *Clinical Journal of Pain*, *13*, 116–137.

Fishbain, D. A., Rosomoff, H. L., & Rosomoff, R. S. (1992). Drug abuse, dependence and addiction in chronic pain populations. *Clinical Journal of Pain*, *8*, 77–85.

Fisher, B. J., Haythornthwaite, J. A., Heinberg, L. J., Clark, M., & Reed, J. (2001). Suicidal intent in patients with chronic pain. *Pain*, *89*, 199–206.

Folstein, M., Folstein, S. E., & McHugh, P. R. (1975). "Mini-Mental State:" A practical method for grading the cognitive state of patients for the clinician. *Journal of Psychiatric Research*, *12*, 189–198.

Fordyce, W. E. (1976). *Behavioral methods for chronic pain and illness*. St. Louis, MO: CV Mosby.

Freedland, K. E., Skala, J. A., Carney, R. M., Raczynski, J. M., Taylor, C. B., Mendes deLeon, C.F., et al. (2002). The Depression Interview and Structured Hamilton (DISH): Rationale, development, characteristics, and clinical validity. *Psychosomatic Medicine*, *64*, 897–905.

Green, C. R., Anderson, K. O., Baker, T. A., Campbell, L. C., Decker, S., Fillingim, R. B., et al. (2003). The unequal burden of pain: Confronting racial and ethnic disparities in pain. *Pain Medicine*, *4*, 277–294.

Guzman, J., Esmail, R., Karjalainen, K., Malmivaara, A., Irvin, E., & Bombardier, C. (2001). Multidisciplinary bio-psycho-social rehabilitation for chronic low back pain. *The Cochrane Database of Systematic Reviews*, *1*, Art. No.: CD000963.

Harstall, C., & Ospina, M. (2003). How prevalent is chronic pain? *Pain Clinical Updates*. Volume XI, No. 2. Seattle, WA: IASP.

Hathaway,. S. R., McKinley, J. C., Butcher, J. N., Dahlstrom, W. G., Graham, J. R., Tellegen, A., & Kaemmer, B. (1989). *Minnesota Multiphasic Personality Inventory 2: Manual for administration*. Minneapolis, MN: University of Minnesota Press.

Hoffman, B. M., Chatkoff, D. K., Papas, R. K., & Kerns, R.D. (2007). Meta-analysis of psychological interventions for chronic low back pain. *Health Psychology*, *26*, 1–9.

Kabat-Zinn, J. (1990). *Full catastrophe living*. New York: Delta Books.

Keefe, F. J., Caldwell, D. S., Williams, D. A., Gil, K. M., Mitchell, D., Robertson, C., et al. (1990a). Pain coping skills training in the management of osteoarthritic knee pain: A comparative study. *Behavior Therapy*, *21*, 49–62.

Keefe, F. J., Caldwell, D. S., Williams, D. A., Gil, K. M., Mitchell, D., Robertson, C., et al. (1990b). Pain coping skills training in the management of osteoarthritic knee pain – II: Follow-up results. *Behavior Therapy*, *21*, 435–447.

Kerns, R. D., Turk, D. C., & Rudy, T. E. (1985). The West Haven-Yale Multidimensional Pain Inventory (WHYMPI). *Pain*, *23*, 345–356.

Liaison Committee on Pain and Addiction. (2001). Definitions related to the use of opioids for the treatment of pain. Retrieved from http://www.ampainsoc.org/advocacy/opioids2.htm.

Loeser, J. D. (2001). Multidisciplinary pain programs. In J. D. Loeser (Ed.), *Bonica's Management of Pain* (3rd ed, pp. 255–264). Philadelphia: Lippincott Williams.

Luthe, W. (Ed.). (1969). *Autogenic training: Vol. 1 Autogenic methods*. New York: Grune and Stratton.

McCracken, L. M., & Dhingra, L. (2002). A short version of the Pain Anxiety Symptoms Scale (PASS-20): Preliminary development and validity. *Pain Research and Managment*, *7*, 45–50.

McMahon, S. B., & Koltzenburg, M. (Eds.). (2006). *Wall and Melzack's textbook of pain* (5th ed.). Philadelphia: Elsevier Churchill Livingstone.

McQuay, H. J., & Moore, R. A. (1997). Using numerical results from systematic reviews in clinical practice. *Annals of Internal Medicine*, *126*, 712–720.

McWilliams, L. A., Cox, B. J., & Enns, M. W. (2003). Mood and anxiety disorders associated with chronic pain: An examination of a nationally representative sample. *Pain*, *106*, 127–133.

Melzack, R. (1975). The McGill Pain Questionnaire. *Pain*, *30*, 191–197.

Melzack, R., & Casey, K. L. (1968). Sensory, motivational, and central control determinants of pain. In D. Kenshalo (Ed.), *The skin senses* (pp. 423–443). Springfield, IL: Charles C. Thomas.

Melzack, R., & Wall, P. D. (1965). Pain mechanism: A new theory. *Science*, *150*, 971–979.

Mersky, H. (1979). Pain terms: A list with definitions and notes on usage. Recommended by the IASP Subcommittee on Taxonomy. *Pain*, *6*, 249–252.

Merskey, H., & Bogduk, N. (Eds.) (1994). *Classification of chronic pain* (2nd ed.). Seattle, WA: IASP Press.

Michna, E., Ross, E. L., Hynes, W. L., Nedeljkovic, S. S., Soumekh, S., Janfaza, D., et al. (2004). Predicting aberrant drug behavior in patients treated for chronic pain: Importance of abuse history. *Journal of Pain and Symptom Management*, *28*, 250–258.

Milton, J. (1910). *Paradise Lost, Books V & VI*. London: Cambridge University Press.

Morley, S. J., Eccelston, C., & Williams, A. (1999). Systematic review and meta analysis of randomized control trials of cognitive behavior therapy and behavior therapy for chronic pain in adults, excluding headache. *Pain*, *80*, 1–13.

National Institutes of Health (NIH). (1995, October). *Integration of Behavioral and Relaxation Approaches into the Treatment of Chronic Pain and Insomnia* (NIH Technology Assessment Statement, pp. 1–34). Washington, DC: Author.

Ng, B., Dimsdale, J. E., Shragg, G. P., & Deutsch, R. (1996). Ethnic differences in analgesic consumption for postoperative pain. *Psychosomatic Medicine*, *58*, 125–9.

Nicholas, M., Molloy, A., Tonkin, L., & Beeston, L. (2000). *Manage your pain*. Sydney, Australia: ABC Books.

Niemisto, L., Kalso, E., Malmivaara, A., Seitsalo, S., & Hurri, H. (2003). Radiofrequency denervation for neck and back pain. *The Cochrane Database of Systematic Reviews*, Art. No.: CD004058.

Onen, S. H., Onen, F., Courpron, P., & Dubray, C. (2005). How pain and analgesics disturb sleep. *Clinical Journal of Pain*, *21*, 422–431.

Ostelo, R. W., Van Tulder, M. W., Vlaeyan, J. W., Linton, S. J., Morley, S. J., & Assendelft, W. J. (2005). Behavioral treatment for chronic low back pain (Review). *The Cochrane Library*, *4*, 1–25.

Pachter, B. (2000). *The power of positive confrontation: The skills you need to know to handle conflicts at work, home and in life*. New York: Marlowe & Co.

Parker, J. C., Frank, R. G., Beck, N. C., Smarr, K. L., Buescher, K. L., Phillips, L. R., et al. (1988). Pain management in rheumatoid arthritis patients: A cognitive behavioral approach. *Arthritis and Rheumatism*, *31*, 593–601.

Pollard, C. A. (1984). Preliminary validity study of the Pain Disability Index. *Perceptual and Motor Skills*, *59*, 974.

Radloff, L. (1977). The CES-D Scale: A self-report depression scale for research in the general population. *Journal of Applied Psychological Measurement*, *1*, 385–401.

Rainville, P., Duncan, G. H., Price, D. D., Carrier, B., & Bushnell, M. C. (1997). Pain affect encoded in human anterior cingulated but not somatosensory cortex. *Science*, *277*, 968–971.

Rainville, P., Hofbauer, R. K., Tomas, P., Duncan, G. H., Bushnell, M. C., & Price, D. D. (1999) Cerebral mechanisms of hypnotic induction and suggestion. *Journal of Cognitive Neuroscience*, *11*, 110–125.

Robinson, M. E., Dannecker, E. A., George, S. Z., Otis, J., Atchsion, J. W., & Fillingim, R. B. (2005). Sex differences in the association among psychological factors and pain report: A novel psychophysical study of patients with chronic low back pain. *Journal of Pain*, *6*, 463–470.

Roland, M., & Morris, R. (1983). A study of the natural history of back pain: Part I. Development of a reliable and sensitive measure of disability in low back pain. *Spine*, *8*, 141–144.

Rosensteil, A. K., & Keefe, F. J. (1983). The use of coping strategies in low back pain patients: Relationship to patient characteristics and current adjustment. *Pain, 17,* 33–40.

Saarto, T., & Wiffen, P. (2005). Antidepressants for neuropathic pain. *The Cochrane Database of Systematic Reviews, 3,* Art. No.: CD005454.

Savage, S. (2002). Assessment for addiction in pain treatment settings. *Clinical Journal of Pain, 18,* S28–S38.

Schultz, J. H., & Luthe, W. (1959). *Autogenic training: A psychophysiological approach in psychotherapy.* New York: Grune and Stratton.

Schwartz, M. S., & Andrasik, F. (2003). *Biofeedback: A practitioner's guide* (3rd ed.). New York: Guilford Press.

Schweitzer, A. (1931). *On the Edge of the Primeval Forest.* New York: Macmillan.

Simon, L., Lipman, A., Jacox, A., Caudill-Slosberg, M., Gill, L., Keefe, F., et al. (2002). *Guideline for the management of pain in osteoarthritis, rheumatoid arthritis, and juvenile chronic arthritis,* APS Clinical Practice Guidelines Series, No.2. Glenview, IL: American Pain Society.

Smith, M. T., Perlis, M. L., Smith, M., Giles, D. E., & Carmody, T. P. (2000). Sleep quality and presleep arousal in chronic pain. *Journal of Behavioral Medicine, 23,* 1–13.

Spitzer, R. L., Williams, J. B. W., Gibbons, M., & First, M. B. (1992). The Structured Clinical Interview for DSM-III-R (SCID): I. History, rationale, and description. *Archives of General Psychiatry, 49,* 624–629.

Sullivan, M. J. L., Bishop, S. R., & Pivik, J. (1995). The Pain Catastrophizing Scale: Development and validation. *Psychological Assessment, 7,* 524–532.

Stewart, W. F., Ricci, J. A., Chee, E., Morganstein, D., & Lipton, R. (2003). Lost productive time and cost due to common pain conditions in the U.S. workforce. *Journal of the American Medical Association, 290,* 2443–2454.

Thorn, B. E. (2004). *Cognitive therapy for chronic pain: A step-by-step guide.* New York: Guilford Press.

Tracey, I., Ploghaus, A., Gati, J. S., Clare, S., Smith, S., Menon, R. S., & Matthews, P. M. (2002). Imaging attentional modulation of pain in the periacqueductal gray in humans. *Journal of Neuroscience, 22,* 2748–2742.

Turk, D. C., & Melzack, R. (Eds.) (2001). *Handbook of Pain Assessment* (2nd ed.). New York: Guilford Press.

Turner, J. A., Holtzman, S., & Mancl, L. (2007). Mediators, moderators, and predictors of therapeutic change in cognitive–behavioral therapy for chronic pain. *Pain, 127,* 276–286.

Udolf, R. (1978). *Handbook of hypnosis for professionals* (2nd ed.). New York: Van Nostrand Reinhold Company Inc.

Valet, M., Sprenger, T., Boecker, H., Willoch, F., Rummeny, E., Conrad, B., et al. (2004). Distraction modulates connectivity of the cingulo-frontal cortex and the midbrain during pain – an fMRI analysis. *Pain, 109,* 399–408.

Van Tulder,M. W., Ostelo, R., Vlaeyen, J. W. S., Linton, S. J., Morley, S. J., & Assendelft, W. J. J. (2000). Behavioral treatment for chronic low back pain: A systematic review within the framework of the Cochrane Collaboration Back Review Group. *Spine, 25,* 2688–2699.

Von Korff, M., Jensen, M. P., & Karoly, P. (2000), Assessing global pain severity by self report in clinical and health services research. *Spine, 25,* 3140–3151.

Von Korff, M., & LeResche, L. (2005). Epidemiology of pain. In H. Merskey, J. D. Loeser, & R. Dubner (Eds.), *The paths of pain 1975–2005* (pp. 339–352). Seattle, WA: IASP Press.

Waddell, G., Newton, M., Henderson, I., Somerville, D., & Main, C. J. (1993). A fear-avoidance beliefs questionnaire (FABQ) and the role of fear-avoidance in chronic low back pain and disability. *Pain, 52,* 157–168.

Ware, J. E., & Sherbourne, C. D. (1992). The MOS 36-Item Short-Form Health Survey (SF-36). *Medical Care, 30,* 473–481.

Webster's New Twentieth Century Dictionary of the English Language Unabridged (2nd ed.). (1983). New York: Simon & Schuster.

Wiffen, P., Collins, S., McQuay, H., Carroll, D., Jadad, A., & Moore, A. (2005). Anticonvulsants for acute and chronic pain. *The Cochrane Database of Systematic Reviews, 3,* Art. No.: CD001133.

Wiffen, P. J., McQuay, H. J., Edwards, J. E., & Moore, R. A. (2005). Gabapentin for acute and chronic pain. *The Cochrane Database of Systematic Reviews, 3*, Art. No.: CD005452.

Wiffen, P. J., McQuay, H. J., & Moore, R. A. (2005). Carbamazepine for acute and chronic pain. *The Cochrane Database of Systematic Reviews, 3*, Art. No.: CD005451.

World Health Organization. (1992). *International statistical classification of diseases and related health problems* (10th rev.). Geneva: Author.

Young, S. (2004). *Break through pain: A step-by-step mindfulness meditation program for transforming chronic and acute pain.* Boulder, CO: Sound True, Inc.

8

Appendix: Tools and Resources

Initial Evaluation Questionnaire

Name _____

Address _____

Phone (_____) _____

Social Security # _____ Date of Birth _____

Sex _____ Marital Status _____

Referring Physician:

Name _____

Address _____

Phone (_____) _____

Reason for referral:

_____ SCS evaluation

_____ Other implantable

_____ Surgical evaluation

_____ Medication evaluation

_____ Cognitive-behavioral program

_____ Psychological intervention

From: B.J. Field & R.A. Swarm: *Chronic Pain*　　　　　© 2008 Hogrefe & Huber Publishers

I. Pain History

Briefly describe pain history (significant events, the approximate dates of those events, and physicians and hospitals):

_____

_____

_____

_____

_____

_____

_____

Treatment History:

Surgery

Dates	Surgeon	Was it helpful?
_____	_____	Yes _____ No _____
_____	_____	Yes _____ No _____

Nerve Blocks

Dates	Physician	Was it helpful?
_____	_____	Yes _____ No _____

Steroid injection

Dates	Physician	Was it helpful?
_____	_____	Yes _____ No _____
_____	_____	Yes _____ No _____

Physical Therapy

Dates	Where	Was it helpful?
_____	_____	Yes _____ No _____
_____	_____	Yes _____ No _____

TNS Unit

Dates	Where	Was it helpful?
_____	_____	Yes _____ No _____

Psychological (relaxation, biofeedback, multidisciplinary)

Dates	Therapist	Was it helpful?
_____	_____	Yes _____ No _____

Chiropractic

Dates	Where	Was it helpful?
_____	_____	Yes _____ No _____

From: B.J. Field & R.A. Swarm: *Chronic Pain*   © 2008 Hogrefe & Huber Publishers

Pain medications past and current:

Medication	Dates	Dosage	Helpful?
_____	_____	_____	Yes _____ No _____
_____	_____	_____	Yes _____ No _____
_____	_____	_____	Yes _____ No _____
_____	_____	_____	Yes _____ No _____
_____	_____	_____	Yes _____ No _____
_____	_____	_____	Yes _____ No _____
_____	_____	_____	Yes _____ No _____
_____	_____	_____	Yes _____ No _____

What makes your pain better? worse? no effect?

	Better	Worse	No effect
Heat	_____	_____	_____
Cold	_____	_____	_____
Bath/shower	_____	_____	_____
Walking	_____	_____	_____
Sitting	_____	_____	_____
Lying down/sleeping	_____	_____	_____
Stress/worry	_____	_____	_____
Exercise/activity	_____	_____	_____
Sexual activity	_____	_____	_____
Reading/television	_____	_____	_____

Pain Pattern:

_____ continuous   _____ comes and goes   _____ brief/momentary

WORSE during a certain time of the day?
      If yes, when? _____

BETTER during a certain time of the day?
      If yes, when? _____

Pain intensity:
Circle the appropriate number: 0 = *no pain*, and 10 = *worst pain imaginable*

AVERAGE pain: 0 1 2 3 4 5 6 7 8 9 10

MINIMUM pain: 0 1 2 3 4 5 6 7 8 9 10

MAXIMUM pain: 0 1 2 3 4 5 6 7 8 9 10

From: B.J. Field & R.A. Swarm: *Chronic Pain*   © 2008 Hogrefe & Huber Publishers

Description of Current Pain:

Symbols:

- - - -	o o o o	x x x x	/ / / /	+ + + +
numbness	pins/needles	burning	stabbing	aching

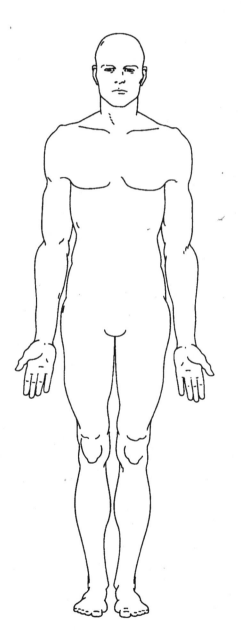
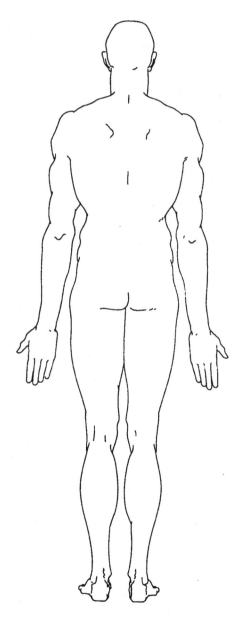

From: B.J. Field & R.A. Swarm: *Chronic Pain*
© 2008 Hogrefe & Huber Publishers

II. Adjustment to Physical Difficulties

Are you currently working?   Yes _____   No _____

    Full-time _____   Part-time _____   Homemaker _____

    If no, how long since you last worked? _____

    Why did you stop working? _____

What is/was your most recent job? _____

Did you enjoy your work?   Yes _____   No _____

Sources of income:

___ Salary	___ Worker's compensation
___ Spouse's salary	___ Personal disability insurance
___ Investment	___ Social security disability
___ Retirement	Other: _____

Pain was the result of injury or surgery? Lawsuits?   Yes _____   No _____

Do you have an attorney at the present time?   Yes _____   No _____

Worker's compensation?   Yes _____   No _____

Describe an average day:

Time up in the morning _____

Daily activities:

    Vacuuming _____   Dusting _____   Laundry _____

    Cooking _____   Shopping _____   Other chores _____

    Yard work _____   Gardening _____

    Hobbies _____

    TV _____ # of hours/day _____

    Reading _____ # of hours/day _____

    Time spent in bed or lying down _____

    Sports _____

    Other recreational: _____

_____

_____

From: B.J. Field & R.A. Swarm: *Chronic Pain*

© 2008 Hogrefe & Huber Publishers

Response of family:

Helpful: _____

_____

Angry: _____

_____

Oversolicitous: _____

_____

Other sources of support:

Religious: _____ Current attendance? Yes _____   No _____

Friends: _____

Socialization: _____

_____

Organizations: _____

From: B.J. Field & R.A. Swarm: *Chronic Pain*   © 2008 Hogrefe & Huber Publishers

III. General Observations

On time? Yes _____ No_____ How late? _____
Previous cancelled or missed appointments? _____
Accompanied by: _____

Pain Behaviors: Yes _____ No_____
        Describe _____

Appearance:
        Height _____
        Weight _____
        Grooming _____
        Dress _____
        Other _____

Oriented? _____
Reliability as historian? Good _____ Poor _____
    Why? _____

Speech: Rate_____ Tone _____ Latency _____
Thought Process: Logical _____ Goal-directed _____
        Circumstantial _____ Tangential _____
Content: Suspicious_____ Perseverative _____
        Other _____
Language and fund of knowledge consistent with education? Yes _____ No _____

Affect: Euthymic _____ Sad _____ Tearful _____ Anxious _____
        Restricted _____ Flat _____ Broad/appropriate_____

Mood: _____
_____

Motivation: _____
Energy: _____
Fatigue: _____

Sleep: Time _____   Fall asleep? _____
        Wakenings? _____   Due to? _____
        Return to sleep? _____   Time up? _____
        Rested? Yes _____ No _____
Medications for sleep: _____

From: B.J. Field & R.A. Swarm: *Chronic Pain*   © 2008 Hogrefe & Huber Publishers

Appetite: Changes? _____   Increase? _____

Decrease? _____   Why? _____

Weight changes? _____

Memory: Changes? _____   Nature of changes_____

Concentration: Changes? _____   Nature of changes _____

Suicidal Ideation: No _____ Yes_____

From: B.J. Field & R.A. Swarm: *Chronic Pain*   © 2008 Hogrefe & Huber Publishers

IV. Psychiatric History

Past and current history:

_____

_____

_____

_____

_____

_____

Psychiatrist: No _____ Yes _____   Name: _____

Medications: _____

Hospitalizations? No _____ Yes _____ # of times _____
Where? _____

Suicidal ideation: No _____ Yes _____
Suicide attempts: No _____ Yes _____ # of attempts _____
Method: _____

Psychological therapy: No _____ Yes _____ # of times _____ duration _____
    Helpful? No _____ Yes _____
    Family history? _____

_____

V. Medical History

Surgeries:
Dates   Procedure

_____   _____

_____   _____

_____   _____

Other medical conditions which have required extended treatment:

_____

_____

_____

_____

Medications other than those for pain relief (include prescribed and OTC):

Medication   For what condition   Dosage

_____   _____   _____

_____   _____   _____

_____   _____   _____

_____   _____   _____

_____   _____   _____

Has any other member of your family suffered from a chronic pain problem?
Yes _____ No _____ If so, who? _____

What type of pain? _____

Substance use:

Do you smoke? No _____ Yes _____ How much _____

Drink alcohol? No _____ Rarely _____ Yes _____ How much? _____ What? _____

History of ETOH use: _____

DUIs: _____

SA Program: _____

Family/work problems: _____

_____

Family history ETOH use: _____

Illicit drug use: No _____ Yes _____ Past _____ Current _____

Marijuana _____ Cocaine _____ Amphetamines _____

Methamphetamines _____ Hallucinogens _____ IV Drugs _____

Other _____

Arrests: _____ SA Program: _____

Family/work problems: _____

Family History: _____

From: B.J. Field & R.A. Swarm: *Chronic Pain*   © 2008 Hogrefe & Huber Publishers

VI. Background and History

Marital status:

Single _____ Married _____ How long? _____ Spouse's occupation: _____

Divorced _____ Separated _____ Widowed _____

Previous marriages _____

Children:

\# _____

Ages _____

Gender _____

Living at home _____ Independently _____

Others in household at the present time?

_____

Family of origin:

Where born and raised?_____

_____

Father: Living _____ Deceased _____

　　　　Occupation: _____

　　　　Current relationship: _____

Mother: Living _____ Deceased _____

　　　　Occupation: _____

　　　　Current relationship: _____

Siblings: Number _____

　　　　Current relationship: _____

Family dynamics:

　　　　Dysfunctional relationships: _____

　　　　Good interpersonal dynamics: _____

　　　　Abuse:

　　　　Verbal _____

　　　　Physical _____

　　　　Sexual _____

From: B.J. Field & R.A. Swarm: *Chronic Pain*　　　　　　© 2008 Hogrefe & Huber Publishers

Education:

High School? Yes _____ No _____ Grade completed: _____
GED? _____
College: _____ Degree: _____
Trade School: _____

Work History:

_____
_____
_____
_____

Recommendations:

1. _____

2. _____

3. _____

4. _____

5. _____

From: B.J. Field & R.A. Swarm: *Chronic Pain*   © 2008 Hogrefe & Huber Publishers

Pain Diary

Fill in pain severity boxes using the numerical scale of 0 to 10 where:

0 -10

no pain   *severe pain*

Week ending: ___/___/___	Mon	Tue	Wed	Thur	Fri	Sat	Sun
Morning – Pain severity							
Afternoon – Pain severity							
Evening – Pain severity							
When my pain was worse, what did I do? Rest? Take medication? Meditate? Stretch? Use heat or ice?							
Physical Factors							
How many hours of sleep did I get?							
Have I been more active than usual?							
Have I stayed on schedule with exercising?							
Emotional Factors							
Do I feel anxious or "stressed"?							
Do I feel depressed or frustrated?							
Do I feel angry or irritable?							
Possible Exacerbating Factors							
Have I visited with friends or family or am I isolating myself?							
Is the weather affecting my pain?							
Am I feeling bored?							

From: B.J. Field & R.A. Swarm: *Chronic Pain*   © 2008 Hogrefe & Huber Publishers

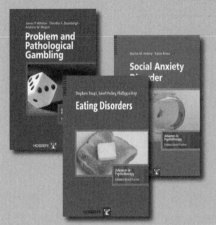
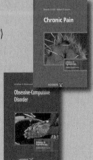

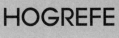

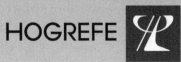